SUGAR LININGS

FINDING THE BRIGHT SIDE OF TYPE 1 DIABETES

SIERRA SANDISON

Table of Contents

Dedication

To every person who is newly diagnosed with diabetes: my guess is that if you are anywhere near as bitter and angry as I was when I was diagnosed, you will not want anything to do with this book right now. I totally get that. I have walked in your shoes. Your mom or some friend probably bought you this book, but the last thing you want to do is spend more energy thinking or learning about this storm cloud that just popped into your life. Maybe it will sit around collecting dust for a while. I know: diabetes sucks. However, my hope for you is that someday, hopefully sooner than later, you can find as many blessings as I have from my disease—maybe even enough to make it all worth it and then some!

To all the parents of children and teens living with T1D: You are incredible. It's not easy being a parent of a child who has a chronic, incurable disease. Yet, you must do so daily. As a consequence, you are among the most compassionate and courageous people I have ever met, and I have nothing but respect and love for all of you! Thank you to Michelle, Bryan, Lisi, Janna, Dan, Lisa, Jeffrey, Lauralyn, Alyson, Tamar, Hallie, Fondra, and so, so, SO many more for being such amazing parents to your kids, and of course, always

having a juice box for me when my teenage forgetfulness and
irresponsibility show themselves. ;)

Of course, to my hero, Nicole Johnson: Without you, I never would
have looked for my sugar linings, nor would I have started out on
this crazy life-changing adventure. Thank you!

Last, but far from least, this book is dedicated to my *favorite* sugar
linings: Hadley, Emma, Evelyn, Tyler, Marie, Madison, McCall,
Avery, Grace, Blair, Vera, Mackenzie, Caroline, Carson, and every
other fellow T1D with whom I have ever crossed paths, even if only
for a moment. Your priceless friendship and presence in my life are
worth every finger poke, every bolus, every bad-blood-sugar-sick-
feeling, and every site change I will ever have to endure throughout
my life.

1: Silver Linings? As In Needles? No Thanks!

Behind every cloud,

there is a silver lining.

~Unknown

I don't know about you, but on the day I was diagnosed with diabetes, I thought this optimistic "Unknown" dude was totally *full* of crap. Who started that proverb? How dare he? He doesn't know what it's like to have to freaking poke and prod myself with needles *all day, every day*! And what about people who have it way worse than I do? Parents who may have lost a child to cancer? Or Holocaust survivors? How could he *possibly* feel like he has the right to tell someone that good things could come from their awful circumstances? Needles are not the kind of silver lines this guy was talking about, but when I was diagnosed, they were the only ones I saw in my future.

More than three years later, I now know that "Unknown Dude" definitely had a point. Diabetes has brought me some amazing opportunities: I now look back at the day the doctor told me I had diabetes and know that being diagnosed with diabetes is one of the most important things to ever happen to me. I am still not a fan of needles, so the term "silver lining" never seemed appropriate: I started referring to the blessings that came from my diabetes as my "sugar linings" instead. And boy, do I have a lot of them now! Perhaps the most obvious one being the #showmeyourpump campaign that helped me reach the top 15 and win the People's Choice Award at Miss America, giving me the chance to proudly wear my t:slim Insulin Pump on national television in front of millions of people. Since then, I have traveled all across the country to speak at diabetes conferences and events, and have been extremely fortunate to meet and spend a ton of time with my awesome, fellow diabetics from all over!

You may also be thinking, "Well, duh, she became Miss Idaho. Of course diabetes worked out well for her. It's easy for her to say there are lots of sugar linings, but what about me or my child?!" While everything to do with my Miss America and Miss Idaho experiences have been overwhelmingly exciting, they aren't my favorite sugar linings. My favorite sugar linings are much more meaningful and, quite honestly, priceless. I wouldn't trade them for the world. Fortunately, they are not unique to me, but rather, are the sugar linings I hear about on a daily basis from other T1Ds from all around the country!

Whether you have been struggling with your storm cloud of type 1 diabetes (T1D) for years, or dealing with a new diagnosis for which the forecast seems bleak or terrifyingly unknown, I am writing this book for you. I aim to offer you hope by not only talking about my unique experience with diabetes, but most importantly, the sugar linings that ring true for any type 1 diabetic who chooses to look for them.

I have faith that you, like so many others have before, will find blessings from this adversity. Wherever you are on your journey with diabetes, I hope that you find strength from your struggles with this disease, and that this book will bring you the hope and courage to do so.

2: The Plan

At first, my extreme thirst didn't bother me. I kind of enjoyed it, actually! I considered myself an overachiever in the area of water consumption: experts suggest that we should drink at least eight glasses of water a day. I, on the other hand, was drinking eight gallons. Bonus points? I think yes! More importantly, I had to leave class at least twice per period to use the restroom and refill the giant water bottle I carried around with me. I wasn't complaining! Until, of course, it started to become inconvenient.

At one point, it became a nightly ritual to pull the coffee table into my room and then cover it with any and every container in the kitchen that could hold water. Soon after that, I found myself falling asleep on the toilet occasionally because it had become too much of a hassle to get out of bed to pee every half hour.

The last straw, however, was one fateful day while I was snowboarding. For those of you who snowboard, you know that, typically, one goes into the lodge once or twice throughout the entire day: once to eat lunch and maybe, *maybe*, once more to go to the bathroom at some point. This fateful Saturday, it felt like I was spending more time in the lodge than I was on the slopes!

Every time I got to the bottom of the hill, I would take off my snowboard to go into the lodge. After having rushed to the bathroom, I refilled my three water bottles, then headed back out to the chairlift. On the rides up, I kept reminding myself that I should invest in the largest camelback I could find for my next ski trip, so maybe the time I would save filling up my water bottles would hopefully add up to an extra run or two. Once or twice, when I stepped off the chairlift at the top, I would quickly find a tree to hide behind to relieve myself, *again*, from the water I had chugged on the ride up.

It was an endless, miserable, inefficient cycle, so I did what any other normal human living in the twenty-first century would do when their body is acting abnormal: I consulted the internet. Of course, Google quickly provided me with the answer I was looking for.

I had figured out what was wrong. So, while still on the chairlift, I called my dad. My dad is a physician, but unfortunately, I had moved out of our house when I turned 18. He probably would have recognized my symptoms sooner if I had still lived at home, but I

wasn't, so I was a little scared to tell him because it might come as
such a shock to him.

"Hello?"

"Dad, I have something to tell you..."

"What is it?"

"Don't be mad."

"Okay..."

"I'm an aquaholic. I need to go to rehab. I'm addicted to water."

. . .

After "admitting I had a problem" to my dad, he kind of laughed
for a second, thinking I was being ridiculous. But once I explained
in more detail how serious my thirst was, he realized what the real
issue was.

I was sure he was wrong. Diabetes? That's insane. I work out almost
every day. Maybe I don't eat extremely healthy food, but what
teenager does? My peers drank way more energy drinks and sodas,
and ate more potato chips and fast food than I would ever dream
of touching. I was tall and skinny. Actually, this was probably the
skinniest I had ever been. Me? Diabetic? No way!

. . .

"Do you believe there is a plan for you life?" The nurse practitioner was just about to plunge a lancet into my finger before my dad interrupted. "If, in a few minutes, we find out that you have diabetes, do you trust that there is a purpose behind it? Do you believe that there is a plan for your life?" My dad is a religious person, but even for someone who isn't, there seems to be some truth to the belief that everything happens for a reason. There are miraculous moments we hear about where someone was in such the right place, at such the right time that it sends chills down our spines. I believe there is a plan for everyone's life. I also believe that good things can come out of bad situations. But I also *knew* that the plan for my life did not include diabetes. That would be ridiculous. "Yes. Sure. Whatever," I thought, as I tried not to roll my eyes as I nodded to appease my dad. I just wanted to prove this whole crazy diabetes theory wrong, so we could finish up this appointment, and I could get on with my diabetes-less life.

You probably know what happened next. In fact many of you have experienced it yourself and are all too familiar with the whirlwind that filled the rest of that day. My blood sugar was in the 500s: the rest of the day was a whirlwind. There was talk about pancreases, insulin, and autoimmune diseases. They told me how this wasn't my fault; and how all day, every day, for the rest of my life, I would be poking and pricking myself with needles. I didn't understand most of what they tried to teach me that day, except for that last part: Needles. *Yay.*

Needless to say, I was beyond upset. I spent the next couple days crying. The sadness then turned into bitterness and anger. I have two—now deceased—relatives with diabetes. Why, out of my gazillions and bajillions of cousins (and two little sisters) was I the only one to develop type 1? What did *I* do to deserve this? Nothing! That's the only answer I could come up with, which made me even more frustrated. Why me? *Why me?!*

I don't remember ever using an orange to practice giving myself a shot like most people do, but maybe that's because sticking a needle into a piece of fruit isn't very traumatizing. However, I vividly remember being in a room surrounded by the nurse practitioner, my parents, and my sister as they watched me screw the needle onto the insulin pen and lift up my shirt. I stopped. Was I really going to stick this sharp piece of metal into my skin? There was no way. Gah. There was also no way that as an 18-year-old I was going to have my mommy give me my shots forever. Would I rather die than give myself a shot? In the moment, I considered it. But no, I had gotten shots before. Plus, this was 2012. The needle was way smaller than the ones my grandpa used for his diabetes back in the '90s. It was also way smaller than the needle the nurse used when I received a flu shot a few months earlier. I pierced my skin and a feeling of nausea hit me as I watched the needle disappear into my body. Ew. It was a creepy concept, but it wasn't painful.

Soon enough, it was over. Some in the room cheered; others stopped holding their breath. Someone congratulated me on my first shot, and it was then I remembered that nothing was "over with." This was just the beginning. The fact that I would have to "do this all day, every day for the rest of [my] life" began to feel real, and not in a good way.

I had spent the last few months getting out of bed to pee several times throughout the night. Tonight, however, it seemed as if the same amount of fluids were leaving my body, but rather than escaping from my bladder, the water escaped through my eyes. The only time I stopped crying following the diagnoses was when my best friend came to visit me. My locker was directly above hers at school, and we had plastered Justin Bieber's face all over the interiors of both our lockers. "Well, Nick Jonas has diabetes," she said. "Maybe someday you'll get to meet him because of it!" I cheered up for a second as we planned to replace all the Bieber pictures with the Jonas Brothers the next day at school. But as soon as she left, my face quickly returned to a wet, swollen state.

A few days later, I was hanging out with my friends and I felt shaky. I don't usually sweat, but I was perspiring like the high school football team did after the state championship game. I wasn't paying attention to that though because of the feeling in my stomach. It reminded me of when a rollercoaster makes a huge drop or when I rode the Hollywood Tower of Terror at California Adventure. Ugh. Had I done something wrong that I felt bad about doing? I got this feeling when I got called to the principal's office and I knew I was guilty of something, or when a friend or boyfriend texted me the dreaded, "we need to talk." I hadn't done anything that I could think of. Why did I feel this way? Maybe it was my blood sugar. I checked, and it was 102. That was the lowest number I had ever seen, but from what I had been told, it was normal and in range. So why did I feel so weird? I changed the lancet and had one of my friends check herself: 82. I should have felt fine at my number! My thoughts were getting foggier and foggier, so I asked my friends to get me some juice. It couldn't hurt. If it didn't solve the problem, I could just bolus a little later. But a few minutes after drinking the juice, my mind started clearing up. I had been so high for so long that in-range blood sugar levels felt like severe lows! Fortunately, I have since grown accustomed to in-range blood sugars. Unfortunately, now I am not sensitive *enough* to lows. Thank god for Dexcom!

• • •

For a long time, I thought the day I was diagnosed with diabetes was the absolute worst day of my *entire freaking life*! Not only did it present endless needles into my daily routine, but it also brought a lot of sickness. No matter how hard I tried, I still had to deal with miserable lows and highs, which would sometimes ruin my entire day. I could do everything right, and somehow my body would still not cooperate.

I don't know about you, but I don't really enjoy doing things that I'm awful at. Diabetes was a huge job and gigantic responsibility— so huge, that I didn't even want to attempt taking care of it. No matter how much effort I put into this disease, I would never have perfect blood sugars, so what was the point of even trying? I don't like failing. It was almost as if I were being forced to pursue a career as a lineman in the NFL: I could pour every ounce of effort and invest every last piece of my soul into doing my best, but at the end of the day, my skinny little feminine frame would never stand a chance.

Obviously, this attitude put me on an emotional and physical roller coaster for the first few months. I didn't have diabetes *burnout*. You can't call it a burnout when there wasn't a fire fueling me to take care of my disease in the first place. Instead, I had immediately given up. (I will refer to this period of burnout from now on though, since it is a common term to describe my attitude and actions towards diabetes.)

I was so jealous of everyone around me. I would be watching TV with my sisters, or sitting in class with my teacher and classmates, and I'd just stare at each of their abdomens trying to guess the exact location where their healthy, functioning islet cells were pumping out insulin. This past weekend, I read Kerri Sparling's (amazing) book *Balancing Diabetes*. (She is also the author behind the blog SixUntilMe.com.) In her book she quotes Manny Hernandez, the cofounder of the Diabetes Hands Foundation. What he said really resonates with me when I reflect on those moments from my early diagnosis spent thinking about other peoples' pancreases, and the pangs of jealousy sometimes I still feel when the thought crosses my mind that my friends never have to worry about the necessary-for-life hormone, insulin. "It reminds me of when I used to scuba dive," he says. "I remember thinking about how much gear you have to wear to dive even a few feet deep, whereas a tiny fish just swims past you with nothing but his God-given body parts." We have to carry around syringes and vials, or insulin pens and needles in our purses and backpacks. We are attached to CGMs and insulin pumps. If we make a mistake, or our body just decides it hates us, we pay the price. Our friends and family never need to give a second thought to how their bodies process the carbs they put into themselves. Why me? Why should I have to?

It was such a huge job to do the work for which my pancreas was supposed to be responsible. What was the point of even trying? When thinking rationally, we diabetics know the consequences of not taking care of our disease. The point of "even trying" is that we all want to live a long healthy life. I want to have healthy pregnancies when I'm older. I don't want to be sick constantly. I don't want to suffer from the complications. I want my dreams to come true. I want to be normal.

As any of you who have experienced burnout know, that fear wasn't enough. Distant fear was not as motivating as the instant gratification I got from saving myself some immediate trouble by skipping a bolus or a finger poke. I was apathetic, indifferent—not scared. And, as I've said before, even when I did a good job of checking and bolusing, I still felt like a failure more often than not. It took me a while to realize that, by definition, being diabetic meant that sometimes (most of the time) my blood sugar would be out-of-range—out-of-range, but not bad.

I recently finished reading Moira McCarthy's excellent book, *Raising Teens with Diabetes*—which, by the way, I recommend to both parents and teens! She makes the very important point that no blood sugar reading is bad. The numbers are never bad; they are just information. I realized that the numbers do not define my success. Instead, whether or not I use the numbers and do the best that I can with the information they provide me with does. If I only patted myself on the back each time my blood sugar was a perfect 100, I would be constantly discouraged and frustrated. The pats-on-the-back need to come every time I bolus, correct, or remember to check my blood sugar, no matter what the number. We all know that regardless of how hard we try, our bodies still don't always cooperate with us. What *does* matter is that we are trying our best!

When I came to the realization that I could be proud of myself—not based on the numbers, but instead because of my honest efforts to control my disease to the best of my ability—I felt much better and found a renewed determination. However, I had an incident that totally knocked me down for a second.

Yesterday, while at my annual eye appointment, the nurse or assistant doing all the pre-check-up stuff before the doctor entered the room was asking me some questions about my diabetes. She asked what my numbers tend to average, and I told her my A1C% (which was one I was proud of). She then continued to ask what my numbers averaged. "On a day to day basis," she asked in a now annoyed tone of voice, "what number usually pops up on the screen of your glucometer when you check your blood sugar?"

I nervously glanced down at my CGM, which was out of her view. The screen showed a roller coaster. I had been at 60 in the middle of the night and corrected. The correction caused it to rise up to 170, where it sat until I had woke up and ate breakfast, which in turn caused it to creep up to 275 before starting its decent back to a "normal" range. Average? It never stays in one place longer than 20 minutes unless I haven't eaten in awhile. Oh, and when I do see a rare straight line of stable blood sugars? I tweet it to the world because it is such a wonderful, uncommon sight!

"Its not that difficult of a question," she continued, when I had hesitated to respond, "When you measure your blood sugar, is it usually 90? 110? 125?"

"I mean…" I stuttered while I tried to form a sufficient answer. "It depends on the time of day, or when the last time I ate was, or if I'm stressed out, or if I am working out, or if I took too much insulin…" I rambled, "I guess it can fall anywhere between 60 and 300 on a usual day… Everyone with diabetes varies that much…"

She looked at me unimpressed, as if I severely neglected my diabetes. "Not everyone," she said under her breath, patronizingly. "Well, maybe you're thinking of type 2 diabetics?" I replied sheepishly. "I'm not as educated on that disease. I do know a lot of other type 1s, and *all* of us have blood sugars all over on a daily basis, unless they are unusually active or eat a very low-carb diet, or maybe have some kind of honeymoon period going on," I babbled on, trying to defend myself. She raised her eyebrows and dropped the subject, knowing that she was right but not wanting to waste her time and energy. For the next thirty minutes or so, I sat in the room finishing up tests and questions, reading lines of letters on a poster hung on the opposite wall, and waiting for the doctor to come in and see me. It gave me plenty of time to reflect on what a rollercoaster my diabetes was: Maybe I should have bolused earlier for breakfast? Should I have lowered my basal rate more throughout the night in order to avoid that low? Ugh! I am such a failure. I didn't know other diabetics usually had perfect blood sugars, but was she right?

On and on my mind went. I was beating myself up. Finally, the eye doctor (a family friend) entered the room. Before trying to figure out the prescription I would need for my glasses, he checked for diabetes-caused damage. The know-it-all, condescending nurse walked in just as he finished. "Wow, you must take great care of your diabetes, Miss Idaho! No retinopathy yet," he said, proudly. She glared at me.

Ha.

I was still a little down in the dumps though. Shortly after leaving, my dad called and asked how it went. Since he is a physician, I asked if he knew any T1Ds for whom it was common to have great blood sugars a majority of the time. He was as confused as I was. "What do you mean?" he asked. "Like, their blood sugars don't fluctuate? That's ridiculous. You know that better than I do." He then went on to add what I had already thought of myself: unless, maybe, if they're eating a low-carb diet and they exercise a lot—which would mean they are far less likely to spike. But the large majority of type 1 diabetics all face a daily struggle to regulate their blood sugar.

Now I felt dumb for letting her make me feel awful about myself.
What did she know? I travel to diabetes conferences every
weekend, meeting hundreds of diabetics at each event. Had I ever
heard one of them say, "I don't know what you guys are
complaining about. Diabetes is easy!" Or, "my child has had
perfect blood sugars for months"? Uhm, no. I absolutely hadn't
heard that come out of anyone's mouth. All of the people I meet
are on the same rollercoaster that I am. My "DiaBesties" send me
daily Snapchats of their CGM screen, usually showing how awful
and crazy their day has been, and wondering how mine was.
Occasionally, I'll see a tweet or Facebook post about how one of
my friends, or maybe a diabetes blogger, had an awesome almost-
straight-line day, but the only reason they post about it is because
it's such a rare and amazing occurrence! None of our blood sugars
are perfect or ideal—that's what it means to be diabetic (like, it's
literally the definition). Despite what that nurse-assistant lady
believes, I do take care of my disease. While my meter or CGM may
not show "perfect numbers," I am trying my very best. That's what
matters.

Now, flashback again to my burnout (if you can call it that):
I hadn't yet had my epiphany about what it meant to succeed at
diabetes. I didn't know many people who had diabetes and had
only heard horror stories about people who suffered from

complications. Also, the local theater company had just put on Steel Magnolias a year before my diagnosis, in which the main character suffered from an exaggerated and terrifying low blood sugar. To make matters way worse, the play ends with the main character dying from diabetes after giving birth. Helpful? Comforting? I think not. (I do enjoy that show though, otherwise.) Again, diabetes was such a huge job, and without having seen or read anything that might provide me with hope, I had decided to give up right away.

My dad calls this my Eeyore phase. While everyone wanted and expected me to be a diabetic Tigger, I was a diabetic Eeyore. As you know, I eventually got through this burnout period of my life. I believe it came to an end due to the culmination of two things:

First of all, my parents have always believed in me. They are constantly telling me that I am independent, smart, and responsible. They "know" I will make the right decision. Is that always true? Of course not! (lol, sorry Dad!) But, nevertheless, they continue to believe. And for the most part, I have transformed to fit the adjectives they label me with. When facing peer pressure, I know that "responsible" is a part of my identity. When it comes to taking initiative, I remind myself that I am independent. When I feel like not doing my homework, I remember that I'm smart, so I better get the grades to prove it.

I have come to be a believer in self-fulfilling prophecies. When my sister was young, my parents had her tested for learning disabilities. After she was diagnosed with pretty much every single learning disability in the book, my parents decided not to tell her about them. Instead, they continued to point out how smart, brilliant, and intelligent she was. They waited until after she had graduated with honors, as student body president no less, to tell her what they had learned when she started elementary school. I think that by instilling these adjectives (negative or positive) in us, we make them part of our identity. No one told my sister that she wasn't cut out for the classroom; she was told she was intelligent and could succeed. She didn't get discouraged. Instead, this motivated her to try harder when something was difficult for her because she didn't know she was "destined to fail", and instead believed she was capable of being successful.

In my case, my parents didn't scold me for being irresponsible with my diabetes. They kept telling me they knew I was responsible and independent, and also knew I would figure it out. Eventually, I believed them. "Yeah!" I thought, "I *am* independent! I *can* do this!" My healthcare provider, Heidi Houser, was also very encouraging and patient with me, and she believed that I could be successful as well. She had seen other people succeed while living with type 1, and she knew that I could too!

Secondly, I heard about Nicole Johnson. Nicole Johnson also has T1D, wears an insulin pump, and happened to be Miss America 1999. Hearing about Nicole and her background influenced me in several different ways, but the way that is relevant to this chapter is when I realized that she had been living with diabetes for almost twenty years. She was fine. Actually, she was more than just fine: she was Miss America! Not only was she taking care of herself and had no complications, but she was also using her diabetes to create a career for herself by inspiring others who lived with the same disease. If Nicole could live well with this disease for twenty years, so could I! She had shown me that it was possible—maybe difficult, but possible.

3: My Hero

After hearing about Nicole Johnson, I quickly made three important decisions that would eventually change my life.

Like, really change my life.

First of all, I was going to take care of myself. Like I said in the previous chapter, diabetes is a big, huge, ginormous responsibility! So big, that I didn't think I could take care of my disease well, even if I tried. So...why should I try? Again, the obvious answer is that, in order to achieve all my dreams, eventually have healthy pregnancies followed by healthy babies, and overall, just have an awesome future, I *had* to at least try.

Once I read about Nicole, I began looking up other well-known diabetics and their success stories. The hope came pouring in. I found out about people who had been living with diabetes for way longer than I had. In some cases, up to seventy years longer!

I also found one of my first sugar linings: I was diagnosed at a time when I had amazing technology to help me handle this disease. If they could live with diabetes for seventy years, starting as far back as the 1940s, then I should definitely be able to do so in 2012! To this day, I am overwhelmingly grateful for things like my beautiful t:slim Insulin Pump and my unbelievably awesome Dexcom, which measures my blood sugar every five minutes without my needing to poke my finger. The job is a lot easier today for me than it has been in the past for people who were diagnosed years before me. Huge props to everyone who was diagnosed before me—who have been kicking diabetes' butt forever!

I also started thinking about all the diabetics who lived ninety-plus years ago, before insulin was discovered in the 1920s. They would have given anything for that lifesaving drug, not to mention a sick touch-screen insulin pump or a continuous glucose monitor! Yet, there I was, not utilizing insulin as best I could. Gah. Sugar Lining #2: Diabetes is no longer a death sentence.

I had learned this lesson before, just in a different way. When I was 14, my family and I moved to Ecuador so that my dad could volunteer in a medical-mission clinic for a year. Up until that point, though I was smart and loved to read, I hated being told exactly what to learn by my teachers, so I was pretty much a straight C student. Luckily, I hadn't hit high school yet, so those C's didn't make it onto any transcript that mattered.

Ecuador changed that attitude. The local kids quickly became some of my closest friends in the world. They worked hard throughout the summer in order to afford their school uniforms for the following year, along with a couple pencils and a notebook. Some of them were unable to come up with the money, which left them to instead work on the farm full-time during the school year. Often among families with many children, once each child reached a certain grade they would drop out of school in order to work to pay for their younger siblings' educations, or, in the worst-case scenario, just to put food on the table while knowing education would most likely never be an option.

Can you say "wake-up call"?

Do you know how cool it is that we can get a high school (and junior high, and elementary) education for free in America? Really, really freaking cool. So I decided that if I had this awesome opportunity right in front of me at home, I needed to take advantage of it to the fullest extent. I was determined to never get less than an A again.

And I didn't, for about six years. During my sophomore year of college, though, I had to take Anatomy and Physiology. It killed me. I got a B and was distraught. However, eventually I realized how much time and energy I had poured into that class trying to get an A. I really, truly tried my best. That's what matters. Getting a B in Anatomy and Physiology was not a failure, because I had put so much effort into learning the materials and doing as well as I possibly could.

My experience with diabetes has been similar. I had the means to take care of my diabetes, but for a while I didn't care. I wasn't motivated. However, seeing Nicole Johnson's example gave me hope! I realized that I am unbelievably fortunate to live in a developed country in the year 2015 for many reasons, but especially because I have access to insulin and a bunch of other amazing tools to make taking care of diabetes easier. I realized that sometimes I will try my hardest to pay close attention to my CGM, bolus early, correct as soon as I don't have insulin on board anymore, etc. Nevertheless, I will still have days where people might consider my blood sugar grade a B-, or even worse. I can't let that discourage me. If I am trying my best, I am succeeding. Everything else is beyond my control, so I can't beat myself up over it. Perfection with this disease (not to mention pretty much everything else in life) is impossible—but that's okay! We need to accept that fact and continue doing the best we can.

The second decision Nicole's example convinced me to make was to finally get an insulin pump.

Let's back up for a second so I can explain something: I wasn't anyone's idea of a beauty queen while growing up. In my elementary school years, I insisted I was one day going to be a paleontologist, entomologist (dinosaur or insect scientist, respectively), or both! I wore overalls everyday, told everyone that I was allergic to the color pink, and wished that professional tree climbing was a realistic back-up to my insect- and dinosaur-related ambitions.

Side note: I vividly remember playing an orphan in the play *Annie*, and having the hair and make-up people think I had taken it upon myself to turn my hair into a rat's nest. Nope. Baths and hairbrushes were also on the list of things I claimed to be allergic too.

As I got older, I became less extreme in my tomboyish-ness, but not any cooler or classier. Braces, unwaxed eyebrows, and perms (an attempt to be low-maintenance) haunt my middle school photos.

High school was less awkward. I traded out the braces for boyfriends, and learned about eyeliner and eyebrow waxing. However, as most teenagers do, I was struggling to fit in. I wanted to be like the cool kids. They didn't have my ginormous hands or gangly body, or get made fun of for being flat-chested. I was still the ever-uncoordinated and slightly annoying Sierra I had always been. I still wanted more than anything to be good at something. I longed to not just be okay at something, but to be known as the best at it! I cheered. I was on dance team. I was in show choir. I played basketball. I ran for student council. I didn't suck at them (okay, maybe I just plain-out sucked at a few of them), but I definitely wasn't a star in any of them. I wanted a talent so bad. I didn't think I had one, and on one of my extra bad days I opened up to a teacher about it. "What are you talking about?" he asked, surprised. "Have you ever looked at your GPA? Compared your test scores to your peers?" He was right. I was definitely still going strong with my straight A's and loving every second of Calculus and Physics. Great. Just great. My talent was being super nerdy? That's *exactly* what I needed to help me climb the popularity ladder.

 Not.

insert un-amused emoji here (with your imagination)

When I was diagnosed with diabetes my senior year of high school, and learned what an insulin pump was, I immediately refused to even consider wearing one. "Are they crazy?" I thought, when my parents and Heidi kept insisting. "I am already pouring all my energy into trying to fit in in high school. Why in the world would I attach a weird medical device to my body, making me feel more different than I already am?!" I, like most teenage girls, spent a lot of time comparing myself to super models. I didn't have the best nose. My hands were not proportionate to my body. And, unfortunately, unlike my breasts (or lack thereof), my tummy was *not* flat. Argh! And now an insulin pump? I HAVE NEVER SEEN A VICTORIA'S SECRET ANGEL, MOVIE STAR, OR ANYONE ELSE GRACE THE RED CARPET WITH A F%#?@!*$ INSULIN PUMP!

Then, I heard about Nicole Johnson. A woman from my church, who happens to direct the Miss Magic Valley pageant (my hometown pageant), is a former Miss Idaho, and has now become a second mom to me, mentioned that there was a former Miss America who also has type 1 and wears an insulin pump. I probably played it cool, but then as soon as I could, I pulled up Google on my phone to find all the information I possibly could about her.

There she was. The beautiful Nicole Johnson. I immediately realized how silly I had been to think that wearing an insulin pump would make me any less beautiful. If any of my peers had a problem with me wearing a medical device, then their opinions weren't really worth worrying about anyways. I slowly realized that this was true for every "flaw" I saw in myself: the big hands, the small breasts, the not-as-flat-as-I'd-like tummy, the glasses I "lost", and the constant presence of a few zits on my face. They were all important parts of Sierra. They were a part of what makes me, me; therefore, they were beautiful, just like my insulin pump was going to be.

Learning to love myself didn't just happen on the outside. I came to understand that being great at math and science is one of the most useful and awesome talents someone could ask for! Most "cool kids" did actually care about their grades, even if it was just to appease their parents. They probably would have even appreciated it if academics came as easy to them as they did for me. I also realized that *everyone* has something that makes him or her feel self-conscious or that they wish they could change about themselves. Even though it can be scary to be different, I know now that I had wasted a ridiculous amount of time trying to fit in. I had tried to hide what made me different. I strove to be less like Sierra and more like the cool kids.

Being different is awesome. If everyone were exactly the same, the world would be horribly, unbearably boring. What if everyone had the same favorite color and wore it everyday and painted every house with it? What if everyone had the same hobby? Or wanted to be the same exact thing when they grew up? I imagine a world full of people dressed in grey, living in grey houses, all knitting, and everyone trying to become a dentist.

Zzzzzzzzzzzzzzzzzzzzzzz...

Not that there's anything wrong with knitting or dentists, but the world works a lot better, and is a lot more interesting, when there are doctors, checkers players, singers, firefighters, and rock climbers in it as well!

Nevertheless, learning to be confident and love myself wasn't an overnight transformation, and I honestly still struggle with it today. Wearing an insulin pump was still a scary concept! Did I really think I was brave enough to wear a machine on me all day, every day? I went back and forth about it for a while, before finally making the decision that, yes, I was going to get an insulin pump.

When I became aware that Nicole had not only made me more comfortable with the thought of wearing a medical device, but also many other things about myself that I had previously wished I could change, I realized how much her example had done for me, my confidence, and my life. With my newfound confidence and understanding of how important it was to love oneself, I made the third decision that Nicole influenced; I would do for others what she had just done for me:

Someday, I was going to wear my new insulin pump on the Miss America stage.

4: Discouraged and Defeated

The moment I made the decision to wear my insulin pump at Miss America, I was sitting next to my best friend, Britanee. I turned to her and just blurted it out:

"Someday, I'm gonna to go to Miss America and wear my insulin pump!"

She stared at me blankly. What was going through her head? I immediately realized how ridiculous that sentence sounded and tried to guess what she was thinking:

A) Insulin pump? What is that? The little machine that Sierra has been so adamant about *not* getting? The medical device thingy that she vents to me about when her parents and doctor try to convince her to wear one?

B) Miss America? Sierra? I mean, I love her, but aren't beauty queens supposed to be graceful, poised, and elegant?

C) Don't you have to have a talent to do pageants, or whatever? What would she do for a talent? Does solving a complex math equation count as a talent for a pageant?

> Lol...she must mean she wants to sit in the audience and watch.

D) All of the above.

D. The answer was definitely D. Not just for Britanee, but it was probably the answer everyone else had as well as I told in them about my new goal the following weeks.

I don't think any of my close friends and family meant to be negative or not to believe in me, but they were used to me being disappointed about bench-warming, not getting the choir solos I wanted, nor landing the lead parts in plays that I was dying for. It wasn't like I was awful at most of the activities I did. I was just never the best. In a beauty pageant, only "the best" ends up with the crown.

The other concern and cause for the lack of support was just that: it was a beauty pageant. Beauty pageants, especially in recent years, have been ripped apart by the media through various accusations, such as objectifying women, placing too much value on beauty, and promoting unrealistic beauty standards. They also have a poor reputation thanks to some young women who have royally screwed up the on-stage question portion of the competition, resulting in entertaining, but painful-to-watch viral videos of the incident quickly spreading across the Internet. With so many messages about how the media is distorting how we should define beauty, the idea of participating in a beauty pageant isn't something that thrills most people, especially the parents of would-be contestants.

SPOILER ALERT

As a side note, before I continue with my story, my experience with the Miss America Organization (MAO) has proved every one of these initial hesitations and assumptions wrong. As you probably know or have guessed, I ended up wearing my insulin pump at Miss America. If I had booked a job as a super model or chosen a pageant system other than Miss America, I would probably not have been allowed to do so. Now that I am more familiar with the history of the Miss America Organization, I know that the women who succeed and participate in the program are incredible. Miss America has truly allowed and encouraged me, along with many women who went before me, to decide upon and portray our own definitions of beauty, rather than force us to fit the mold society and the media pressure us into thinking beauty should look like. Nicole Kelley, Miss Iowa 2013, was born with only one arm, and was absolutely breathtaking on the Miss America stage. Olivia McMillan, Miss America's Outstanding Teen 2015, was open about sharing her weight struggles. As she competed, the entire audience made it clear that her relatable, genuine, and inspiring message about *body image and self-esteem had won their hearts, and that Olivia had what our country now values in a role model for our teens. There are other ways, too, in which former Miss America contestants and winners have touched hearts across the nation. Heather Whitestone, Miss America 1995, was the first deaf woman to win the national title. Alexis Wineman, Miss Montana 2012, was the first woman with autism to compete for the Miss America title. All of these women and many more have shown me that being beautiful means being the best Sierra I can possibly be. It does not mean I should spend my energy trying to look like someone else, whether that be a flawless movie star or the popular girl at school. We have been told that beauty means fitting into one narrow mold, when the truth is that the more diverse we are, the better! While competing in the Miss America Organization, I met hundreds of amazing young women, all of whom are different—but every single one of them is beautiful in their own way. Thank you, MAO, for encouraging me to be myself, to be different, and to not waste my time trying to fit in while I could be standing out and making a difference instead! As for objectifying women, the Miss America Organization has done nothing but empower me and provide me with amazing opportunities. The work that goes into preparing for a pageant, such as community service, public speaking, keeping up-to-date on current events, maintaining a healthy, fit lifestyle, etc., makes up 99% of "my pageant experience." The other 1% is the* one or two nights a year I put on an evening gown, some make-up, and a pair of high heels and get on stage! There is absolutely nothing to be ashamed of if a woman enjoys getting dressed up. I love pageant night! But there is so much more to the Miss America Organization than one might guess from the outside. There is nothing innately wrong with beauty, or feeling beautiful, but it is important that we understand that beauty isn't the most important aspect of life, nor should the label "beautiful" be exclusive to only the tall, skinny, symmetrical women on the planet. Because of the Miss America Organization, I overcame my fear of public speaking. I realized the importance of staying informed and passionate about what is going on in my community, country, and the world. I am a leader of tomorrow, and without knowing what problems we face in our future, I will not be equipped to find their solutions. Because of MAO, I also entered my freshman year of college with the determination to make sure I still made time for exercise and to research the importance of nutrition. Most importantly, the Miss America Organization taught me to love myself. Learning to not only tolerate but also to love the things that made me different and to think of my insecurities as things that made me unique were the most empowering lessons anyone could have ever taught me. I hope my decision to wear my insulin pump proudly has shown both diabetics and non-diabetics to be proud of who they are, and to

stop trying to hide what makes them different and to own their
differences proudly instead.

Now, back to before I learned all that awesome stuff:

My friends and family never discouraged me from competing in a pageant; they just weren't totally stoked about the idea. Understandable. But hey, if I was going to get an insulin pump because of it, Miss America was an activity they would be supportive of.

I decided that solving a math problem was probably not going to fly with the audience or judges, so I decided to try and sing. I was, and am still, no Beyoncé, but I am [usually] not painful to listen to (as long as there are no high notes).

So, a few months after making the decision to compete, I entered the Miss Magic Valley program for the first time.

Aaaaaaaand...guess what happened? :D

I ended up finally finding my calling in life; I was a beauty pageant prodigy! The judges gushed. They swore that within a year I would easily, beyond a doubt, become Miss America.

Just kidding. I lost.

I did have a blast though. The girls were awesome, kind, fun, intelligent, and passionate about their community service platforms (contrary to my expectations, which, of course, were based on *Toddlers and Tiaras* and *Miss Congeniality*). I learned a lot about how to hold myself and improve my posture. I had a rough interview, but of course, that just helped me know what to prepare for interviews in the future, and further crushed my preconceived ideas about pageants. How do I, an 18-year-old girl, suggest we better our economy? Geez. The winner has to know that? No one taught me anything about that in high school.

My friends and family insisted that I rocked it and looked beautiful. I started to doubt their sincerity when Brit suggested that "maybe… [I] should become a famous math person who, like, wears an insulin pump while solving calculus problems…and inspire little kids that way?".

Nope. I was determined. Math was awesome, but I was going to wear my insulin pump on the Miss America stage.

I worked really hard for a few months, and then went to a nearby town to compete at their [very small] pageant, which had four other contestants, aside from myself.

Aaaaaaand…guess what happened this time?

I won.

For reals.

I'm serious this time.

I WAS GOING TO COMPETE AT MISS IDAHO!!!!!!!!!!!!!!!!!!!!!!!!!!!!!!!

Dear Mrs. Corpron, Mrs. McCallister, and Mrs. Silvers,

I thought this would be a good time to apologize to my former-English teachers for the times I say "gonna" or "kinda"; puuuuut extra vowels in my words in order to be dramatic or build suspense; my incomplete, abrupt or even one-word "sentences"; the sixty extra exclamation points above and below; and any other grammatical errors that I feel help me better express my emotions/be myself (an eternal child and partial drama queen) in my writing. Just be glad that I'm not allowed to put emojis in here.

But really: I WAS ACTUALLY GOING TO MISS IDAHO!!!!!!!!!!!!!!!!!!!!!!!!!!!!!!!!

The way the Miss America Organization works is that you compete at a local pageant—for example, Miss San Francisco, Miss Los Angeles, or Miss Boise. If you win the local pageant, you are then qualified to compete at the state level, such as Miss California or Miss Idaho. And, of course, if you win a state title, you then advance to Miss America.

Step one of wearing my insulin pump at Miss America was officially complete: I was Miss Pocatello and headed to Miss Idaho. However, I knew the next step was going to be much more difficult.

The next summer, I packed up and headed up to Boise for Miss Idaho week! I was so excited. It exceeded my expectations. The girls were all so unbelievably awesome, and many of them have become some of my closest friends. We had the opportunity to participate in fun service projects throughout the week, to stay up late every night talking and laughing (because having a slumber party with that many girls is a rare and precious occasion), and of course, we never missed a chance to debate politics over lunch

Miss Idaho week starts off with all the contestants moving into the dorms we stay at. Immediately after everyone is settled, we start rehearsals, which, aside from service projects and meals, take up the majority of our time until the competition officially starts. The competition itself takes place over the course of a few days. On Thursday, we have our private interviews with the judges. On Friday night, all of the contestants compete. At the beginning of the night on Saturday, all the young women stand on stage and the emcee reads the names of the final eleven contestants who will advance to the next round. The top eleven step forward before they rush backstage to get ready to compete all over again. The remaining women are eliminated. Later, the judges make another cut, leaving only a top five. After those finalists answer a final on-stage question, the emcess reads off the runners-up, and, finally, announces the winner.

My first year at Miss Idaho, there were just eighteen girls competing. "That makes it easy to get into the top eleven," I told myself. I knew I wasn't the best—there were girls who had been competing at Miss Idaho for four, five, or even six years. But still, being in the top two-thirds this year wouldn't be much of a challenge. My interview went pretty well, and so did my eveningwear and swimsuit portions. I messed up a little in talent, but doesn't everyone?

As it turned out, on Saturday night, once they finished listing-off the top eleven, I remained standing at the back of the stage among the rest of the bottom seven.

Ouch.

I was upset. But then I had some Olive Garden breadsticks delivered backstage and everything was okay again.

Kinda.

I will never underestimate Olive Garden breadsticks' (or pizza's, or chocolate's, or cheesecake's) ability to improve unfortunate circumstances, but I also know they can't always completely fix every situation. They can't bring a lost loved one back to life. They can't make your high school sweetheart love you again after a break up. They also won't change the fact that you didn't make top eleven at the Miss Idaho pageant, and not making the top eleven meant my chances of ever actually winning Miss Idaho in the future became pretty slim. I finally saw the reality that my friends and family saw: I was probably never going to wear my insulin pump at Miss America.

@%#&$*?@$!@*$#

Did I give up? "Of course not," you say! Well, actually, yeah. I kind of did. Up until then, I had actually never worn my insulin pump in a pageant. My reasoning was that at Miss America, unlike Miss Magic Valley or Miss Idaho, there would be tons of media helping the public get to know the contestants better. That is how I, and the world, learned about Alexis Wineman's having autism and Nicole Kelley's story of being born with only one arm. Without the media explaining why I had a little machine attached to my hip, I thought my efforts would be pointless. How were they supposed to understand my message without me explaining it to them? I decided to reevaluate my goal, and make a more realistic one: I was going to go back to Miss Idaho, once more, so that I could wear my t:slim on stage in a pageant. I wanted to prove to myself that I was brave enough to do so. "After all," I thought, trying to justify my now-downgraded goal, "it will actually take more bravery to wear it without being able to explain myself first, right?"

The other problem I now faced was that, initially, I knew that everyone had his or her own "pump." The pump was a symbol of the things that *every single one of us* has that make us feel different and, therefore, insecure. And while I knew that, I also knew that wearing my insulin pump would be most meaningful to other people with type 1 or, at least, other people who also wear medical devices. With a national audience of millions watching Miss America, there were bound to be a lot of people with insulin pumps and other medical devices watching! However, with the small, limited audience at a local or state pageant that isn't broadcast on even local TV stations, the chances of even one person with a medical device being in the audience were slim.

Despite all these disappointing considerations that were stuck in my head after making the decision to lower my goal, the thought of not competing with my insulin pump ever—*at all*—was even more depressing after my having determinedly dreamt about doing so for so long.

Over the next year, a lot of big, awesome things happened. I will try to sum them up quickly, since they don't directly pertain to my insulin pump. Right after Miss Idaho, I competed again to be Miss Magic Valley. This time, I won! I then left to spend the last three weeks of my summer vacation in Cambodia, volunteering with several schools all over the country, as well as checking *Angkor Wat* and *Riding an Elephant* off my bucket list. I fell in love with a few precious little children there and was devastated to leave them. One of the most moving parts of the trip was visiting the prisons and killing fields from the Cambodian Genocide carried out by the

Khmer Rouge. If you are not familiar with the event, it is basically Cambodia's version of the Holocaust. Much like the lessons I learned during my time in South America, my trip to Cambodia gave me a new outlook on the world.

I grew up a lot during the following months. I gained leadership skills by partnering with my younger sister, Hailey—who had since joined me in doing pageants—on her platform. She started an organization called Possibilities that puts on sports camps for students with cognitive and physical disabilities. It gave them the opportunity to participate and excel at extracurricular activities they were normally excluded from. It had an amazing effect on the community by connecting the athletes with their peers who volunteered. It gave them an identity beyond the hurtful and politically-incorrect identities their peers had previously attributed to them: "Grace the Down Syndrome girl," "Derek is special needs," and so on. Now, James was funny; Abby was a great volleyball player; Cooper loved to dance. One athlete from our camp even went on to make the high school's varsity basketball team!

One day, while Hailey was helping out in the special education classroom, she asked the students what they would do if they knew they wouldn't fail. She expected huge, crazy ideas, but one girl's response surprised her: "I would try out for the cheer team like you, Hailey!"

Cheerleading and other extracurricular activities had always come easily for us. Hailey realized that she had been taking these activities for granted: many of her peers weren't able to participate in them, whether it was due to having a disability, not being able to afford them, or both! She also realized that while extracurricular activities in her mind were mostly just for fun, they had shaped her identity and helped her discover who she was and what she had a passion for. Most importantly, they built character and taught her how to work hard. She quickly realized how unfair it was that her friends were missing out on the fun and important activities she had enjoyed throughout her entire life. She also realized it would be a fairly easy problem to fix. "Ally's greatest wish is to be a cheerleader? Let's make it happen!"

Soon, she had organized a basketball and cheer day camp, which allowed the students to get out of classes for the day and, instead, spend time fulfilling their dreams of dribbling down the court and cheering on the sidelines. In the evening, the entire community was invited to watch a game, as well as the joy that spread across the faces of both the athletes that racked up points on the scoreboard and the cheerleaders that showed off their cartwheels at halftime.

I was at a point in my diagnosis that I desperately wanted to take a break. I obviously couldn't stop taking insulin and testing my blood sugar, but with all the activities I had been doing for my diabetes awareness platform for Miss Idaho, I began to feel as if I were letting diabetes define me and allowing it to completely take over my life (I will discuss those feelings in greater detail later). This happened at about the same time Hailey started Possibilities, so I decided to take a break from my diabetes activities and to, instead, change my platform and jump on board with her new project.

One day, after a soccer camp was wrapping up, we were taking pictures and one of the athletes loudly asked me about my insulin pump. It never feels good when someone points out an insecurity of mine, so at first I was a little frustrated and attempted to change the subject. She persisted though, and I eventually explained what diabetes is and how I had to wear my t:slim so it could constantly give me the medicine I needed. She continued the conversation by asking some serious, but honest questions, which were uncharacteristic of her loud, silly personality:

"Do you ever feel different and wish you weren't?"
"Have you ever been bullied because of it?"
"What do you do when people are mean?"

After that day, that athlete stayed by my side at every camp Hailey and I held, claiming that I was her best friend because I knew what it was like to be different.

That was the moment I realized how much we could relate to each other, even though our struggles were different. I had tried to step away from my diabetes, but what I had learned from it continued to follow me everywhere. I decided I was okay with that. I also felt better about not being able to wear my insulin pump at Miss America. She wasn't diabetic, so maybe the non-diabetic audience at Miss Idaho would also understand and benefit from my message more than I thought they would.

In January, I left for Europe, where I spent the next five months backpacking alone around twelve different countries. I can't even begin to name the lessons I learned there. First of all, being alone for so long in a strange place made me feel extremely independent. It forced me out of my comfort zone and helped me meet new people from all different backgrounds and cultures. It introduced me to new worldviews and people who think differently than I do. I learned many things about history that I did not learn in high school, which, much like the experiences I had while living in a third world country, taught me to appreciate the things we take for granted, such as freedom of speech and religion, and obviously the advances we have made in science and medicine. I remember one stomach-churning incident while I was on an educational tour, learning about the witch hunts (and tortures that followed them), and all of a sudden a wave of gratefulness swept over me as I realized how extremely fortunate we are to have the right to a fair trial by jury.

(I remember that night at dinner saying, "Dear God, thank you for this food. And, oh, and thank you for the Sixth Amendment. Amen.")

But seriously, we are so fortunate.

In addition to my exposure to new cultures and interesting historical information, the then current Miss Idaho challenged me to fulfill a New Year's Resolution. She had asked all the local titleholders to make a resolution, and proposed we all hold each other accountable for keeping our resolutions. I knew that on January 1st I was getting on a plane to Italy. As the other girls made their vows to cut down on junk food and put in more hours at the gym, I was thinking, "screw that!"

There was no way I was going to worry about cutting back on carbs in Italy! I was not going to skip a weekend wine-tasting tour through Tuscany in order to spend some time at the gym. Pass on the French crepes in Paris? No thanks. Nope. No, no, no.

So, instead, I decided that my New Year's Resolution would be to read at least one book per month in 2014. I have successfully followed through with (and have far exceeded) that goal, continuing it to this day, but my time in Europe was extra full of train, bus, and plane rides where my reading time seemed infinite!

Finally, I came home from Europe and had three months to hit the gym, master my talent, and turn in my paperwork for Miss Idaho.

In my Miss Idaho interview, almost every single lesson I had learned that year came up in my discussion with the judges: the stories about the athletes I work with at Possibilities' camps, how Europe had made me more independent, how I admired Eleanor Roosevelt and had just finished her 500-page autobiography, and how Sheryl Sandberg's book, *Lean In*, helped shape my feminist views.

The reason I felt it was important to provide details about the year between my not making top eleven and when I won Miss Idaho is that I want you to understand that winning Miss Idaho didn't just happen to me. I worked hard to go from the very bottom to winning in just one year. Whether your goal is to become Miss America, fly to the moon, or become President of the United States, believing you can do so is important, but there is still a lot more involved in reaching the goals you set for yourself. Work hard; do everything with passion and compassion; learn as much as you can about yourself, the world, and the topics that interest you and that pertain to your goals. Do interesting, adventurous things that people want to hear about.

Now, let's get back to Miss Idaho week. As I have already said, my interview went well. That part I loved! Now it was time to go on stage. I finished my make-up, unrolled my curlers, and clipped my t:slim Pump to my pants pocket for the opening number.

All of a sudden, I was terrified. My insulin pump suddenly seemed *a lot* bigger than it usually did. I was reminded again that the audience had no idea what this strange thing attached to me was, let alone the message I was trying to send with it! What had I been thinking? This was stupid. I was stupid. Ugh.

No. No I wasn't. This may not have turned out as inspiring as I had originally intended it to when I thought I could make it to Miss America, but I was still going to do it. I didn't get into pageants to win a crown or to give my peers a reason think more highly of me. I didn't do it to add to my resume or because I loved hair, make-up, and heels. I did it because I wanted to make a difference by wearing my insulin pump on stage. At this point, I didn't know if it would even have an impact, but I knew that if I decided to give up now, I would always wonder if it would have.

I walked out of the dressing room, telling myself not to worry. No one was going to notice. It wasn't a big deal. No one was going to notice!

"Seriously," I repeated in my head as I joined the rest of the contestants behind the curtain, "no one is going to notice."

5: Getting Noticed

There were about ten minutes until show time. I could hear indecipherable murmuring from the audience. Was anyone staring at me? Or, at my insulin pump? No. As I scanned the room, I saw nineteen other young women chattering away, hyped up on adrenaline, nerves, and excitement. The crew was busy getting tech stuff prepared and running around like headless chickens in their black clothes. There was a little girl standing over by the...

Wait, what? What is she doing back here? Not that I would normally care, but she was staring at me!

No, wait.

She was staring at my *insulin pump*.

At least, it felt like it. "Maybe I'm overthinking," I reassured myself again. I turned away and quickly tried to jump into a conversation with a nearby group. A few moments later I glanced nervously towards her. "She's still looking!" I screamed inside my head, as our eyes met. "NO! Not eye contact. How did I let that happen? ARGH!"

Eye contact can be mistaken for an unspoken invitation of sorts. It wasn't.

And then, it came. The dreaded question:

"What is that?" she asked, pointing at my insulin pump.

I turned to head towards the dressing room. "Kids!" I thought, "Why don't they have filters? Why are they so curious about people who are different? Can't they be polite? And for heaven's sake, *why* did she have to ask right at *this* moment when I am terrified out of my mind?"

"Wait!" she called to regain my attention, "Is that an insulin pump?"

So…she knew what it was? Okay, so the comment was a little more understandable now. "Yes…" I responded, hesitantly. "Oh sweet! I'm diabetic, too! I've been looking for you," she replied. "Whoa!" I replied, shocked. "That's awesome!" This changed everything. We proceeded to discuss diabetes, when we were diagnosed, etc. She introduced herself, and said her name was McCall. She was Miss Idaho's Outstanding Preteen, which was why she was allowed to hang out back stage.

Finally, I asked, "What kind of pump do you have? Do you wear a t:slim too?" She got quiet. "Oh…" she mumbled, "I don't have one. I'm just in sixth grade. I don't know what my friends would say if I, well…you know, had a machine attached to my body. It's a little weird."

Holy crap. This was beyond awesome. I mean, of course, it saddened me that she felt that way, but *this was my chance*. Forget about going to Miss America! That's not really what I wanted anyways. My sole purpose when starting pageants was to be Nicole Johnson for others. Even if I only made a difference in one person's life, that was enough for me! And here she was: not only was there a little girl with diabetes, but she was also a girl who didn't feel confident about wearing an insulin pump, and she would be watching tonight as I wore mine on stage for the first time. She was like the 18-year-old Sierra Sandison about to hear about Nicole Johnson for the first time. All of my fear, anxiety, and hesitation were suddenly gone—and just in time! The emcee had begun to welcome the audience, and the curtain was about to open.

I competed that night with all the confidence in the world. Who cared about what the audience thought? Who cared about the judges? Not me, that's for sure! All that mattered was the little beauty queen who had her eyes glued on me.

When the first night of competition ended, McCall ran up to me, jumping up and down and talking a million miles per hour. "Guess what?!" she exclaimed. "I am getting an insulin pump! I talked to my mom, and I'm going to get an insulin pump!" (Or, as I heard it, "IMGETTINGANINSULINPUMP! OMGOMGOMG! ITALKEDTOMYMOMANDIMGONNAGETANINSULINPUMP!")

She quickly darted off to tell her other friends who had come to watch. Immediately after she disappeared, a beautiful blonde woman approached me. She introduced herself as McCall's mom and, in tears, explained what a controversial issue the insulin pump had been in their family for as long as she could remember. She said that she had begun to doubt if McCall would ever agree to wear one, and she definitely never imagined a day where she would be jumping up and down, full of excitement at the thought of getting a pump.

My heart jumped out of my chest. I had done it. My impact had been way more effective and came far more quickly than I could have ever imagined in my wildest dreams! I was in complete shock. Was this real life?

"Honestly Sierra," I told myself, "you probably won't become Miss Idaho tomorrow." And I knew that I was completely okay with that. I wasn't chasing after a crown, I just wanted a chance to make a difference or have an impact on someone else's life. I couldn't believe it had just happened. Unlike birthdays, where you have big expectations for how wonderful you will feel when you are one year older, and then totally feel exactly the same when midnight strikes, this actually did feel incredible. I just achieved one of the most difficult, but also most rewarding goals of my life to date: I had done for McCall what Nicole had done for me.

In my heart, I had won. Maybe I hadn't won the prize that the rest of the women were aiming for by coming to Miss Idaho, but to me, it was the only one that mattered. I didn't want the crown, I just wanted to know I had made a difference in someone else's life.

This week could not possibly get any better.
Or could it?

6: "And The New Miss Idaho is…"

I was still on cloud nine the following evening. It was Saturday night, a.k.a., finals night. My fellow contestants and I were lined up across the stage in a giant semi-circle, awaiting the emcee to read off the list of the top eleven finalists who would move on in the competition. It was no longer my goal. I was ready to go back to my normal life, have my dad bring my Olive Garden breadsticks backstage again, and and continue to reflect on the fact that I had actually achieved my goal, and how all of my hard work had truly paid off. I couldn't believe it…

"Contest number nineteen, Sierra Sandison!" one of the emcees exclaimed.

"Whoa, what?" I snapped back to reality as I made my way up to the front to join the rest of the girls whose names had already been called to advance to the top eleven. I barely had time to process anything, as we were quickly whisked off stage in order to rapidly get ready to compete all over again.

"Wow," I thought, "I improved from last year! That's awesome. Breadsticks can wait, I guess." I definitely wasn't complaining. And I was making McCall proud! We had taken a picture together the night before, and she had spent her Saturday morning getting it developed, framed, writing a card, and also making a magnet with my picture that said "Miss Idaho 2014" on it. Ha. No pressure. At least now I knew that her "hero" wouldn't be standing in the back, getting eliminated immediately. That was a relief.

After repeating all areas of the competition again, the top eleven made another semi-circle across the stage. The emcees began to read off the names of the young women who would now advance to the top five. Again, to my surprise, they called my name. "Contestant number nineteen, Sierra Sandison!"

"Wow. Wow. Wow." I thought, as I stepped forward, exchanging a hug with the young woman whose name had been called before mine (who, by the way, was the first runner-up in 2013 and is one my great friends).

Once they had named the last young lady who had made the top five, we passed a microphone down the line, and were each asked one final on-stage question. After that, we headed backstage to wait for the judges to tally up their scores and make their final decisions.

Once we were finally allowed back on-stage, we spent about fifteen minutes giving away awards, such as non-finalist interview, rookie talent (for a girl who is competing for the first time), the fundraising award, the environmental scholarship, and so on. Finally, the top five were asked to step forward.

As we held hands, I had no idea what to expect. One of my friends who had competed with me last year, not making the top eleven then either, had worked her butt off for the last twelve months, just as I had, and now stood with me among the top five. A second finalist had only made top eleven the previous year; a third had made top five twice before and, as I said, was first runner up in 2013. The fourth girl had never competed at Miss Idaho before this year, but she was one of the most talented, brilliant, and hardworking women I have ever met. And then, there was me.

They started calling off names.
"The fourth runner-up in the Miss Idaho competition is…"

Not me.

"Your third runner-up for the year of 2014 is…"

Again, not me.

"The second runner-up goes to…"

Still, not me.

I turned to face the other girl who remained; we held hands in the traditional way that the top two finalists always do as they await the results. There was no way. This was insane. What was happening?

The emcee dragged out the job description of the first runner-up for a little too long. "The first runner-up is a very important position. If for some reason Miss Idaho should relinquish her title during the year, the first runner-up will take her place."

Et cetera, et cetera. Yeah, yeah, we know!

"The first runner-up, and the winner of a $4,000 scholarship, award plaque, and entry fee to the National Sweetheart Pageant (a pageant that all the first runners-up from the Miss America state pageants are invited to compete at) is…"

Not. Me.

Holy $#!%*@. The audience erupted.

"...that means," he continued, "that your new Miss Idaho, for the year 2014, is...Sierra Sandison!"

What the heck just happened?! To this day, I cannot, for the life of me, remember anything that happened after that moment. At some point, I remember looking out into the audience and screaming over and over again, "BRITANEE! I AM GOING TO MISS AMERICA! WITH MY INSULIN PUMP! I'M GONNA WEAR MY INSULIN PUMP AT MISS AMERICA!"

Apparently, I was so out of it that at some point that my crown came loose and crashed to the ground. I didn't notice, so I just kept walking around, hugging and talking to people. I've been told that a few of the girls quickly grabbed the crown and the scattered jewels, and pinned it back on my head with their own bobby pins. The only reason I even know this happened is that at about 2 am, after I had gotten back to my hotel room, the second runner-up messaged me on Facebook and asked me how my crown was. Confused, I responded that it was beautiful! She then asked, "oh wonderful! I was so scared that it was broken." "What?" I thought.

"Why would it be broken?" I asked her. She told me it had fallen, and I ran across my hotel room to check it. Sure enough, it was bent and still missing some jewels. It wasn't a huge issue. We sent it in for repairs, and it was fixed and returned promptly. However, to this day I wish I could remember that moment because the pictures of the other girls pinning the crown back on my head melt my heart!

I wish I could remember more of that night for another obvious reason: it was the most amazing, monumental, incredible night of my life so far. I had thought the night before was the highlight of my life and that the weekend couldn't get any better than it already was. Little did I know, even more exciting events were in store!

7: #ShowMeYourPump

On Friday night, following the first round of competition, I had posted a picture of McCall and me on Facebook, along with the story of how Nicole had inspired me and, in turn, how I had been able to give McCall the confidence to wear an insulin pump. My pump was not visible in the picture, but diabetics who were friends with McCall and Nicole (who were both tagged) saw it and commented, asking me to post a photo of myself where they could see my insulin pump.

A few days after winning the title of Miss Idaho, I received the CD of pictures from the photographer. I scrolled through and decided upon a picture from the lifestyle and fitness competition, because the pump was blatantly obvious: it was clipped to the side of my swimsuit. It was also the most vulnerable picture—and wearing a medical device proudly was a vulnerable thing to do. I posted it, along with the following caption:

"There it is. I would never have dreamt of posting a swimsuit picture on social media, but diabetics from all over the country have been asking to see me and my insulin pump on the #MissIdaho2014 stage. Honestly, it is terrifying walking out on stage in a swimsuit, let alone attached to a medical device. My message to everyone, diabetic or not, is that we all have something that doesn't "measure up" to the beauty standards set by the media--and that is okay! It does not make you any less beautiful. We also all have obstacles, challenges, and trials. Diabetes turned my life upside down when I was first diagnosed. Don't let your challenge hold you back or slow you down. Use it not only to empower yourself and grow as an individual, but also to serve and influence other people as well.

"With that said, I have faced my fear of proudly showing my insulin pump! Now I want to see YOURS! Post your photo on social media (Instagram, Twitter, Facebook—and make sure it is shared publically so I can see it) with the hashtag #showmeyourpump! The nationwide support from my fellow diabetics this weekend has been AMAZING! I can't wait to see more of you guys!

"This is not limited to just girls, or to people with pumps--I want to see YOU and whatever your daily battle with diabetes looks like.

"All my love,

Sierra

Miss Idaho 2014"

Honestly, I was expecting to receive my average of about a hundred likes per post. I worried that most people would either be too insecure or just not take the time to post a picture of themselves showing their pumps. So I went about my day and kind of forgot about the post.

As you may know, I came back to my computer later that night and was shocked to see that the picture had been both liked and shared *thousands* of times: it had gone viral. Soon, #showmeyourpump was trending on Twitter. My social media exploded with new followers, and people tagging me in pictures. As of today, if you search #showmeyourpump on Instagram, over 6,000 pictures will pop up (and that doesn't include the pictures from Instagram accounts that are set to private). We have estimated that with all social media outlets combined, as well as trying to take into account the pictures that are hidden due to privacy settings, that over 25,000 #showmeyourpump pictures have been posted since the day the hashtag started trending.

I received letters, messages, emails, and pictures, not only from people across the United States, but from people in over thirty-five different countries as well! Over the following weeks, my social media newsfeeds were overflowing with pictures of people with their insulin pumps and other diabetes supplies. However, one of the things that touched me the most was also seeing pictures of children with hearing aids, prosthetics, glass eyes, feeding tubes, and scoliosis back and leg braces. My message wasn't exclusively aimed at diabetics, but every single person I could possibly reach. It meant so much to me that people were understanding the message I wanted to convey: no matter who you are, there is something that inevitably makes you feel different or self-conscious. Do not hide it! It is part of what makes you, you! Be proud of it and celebrate it. It makes you unique!

Many have told me that my story, as well as the #showmeyourpump campaign, really touched and inspired them. However, I feel like the person who it has impacted the most has been me. I wish every single person who has any ounce of insecurity in themselves or from their diabetes could have also been on the receiving end of all of the messages, pictures, letters, and stories that I was getting during my first few weeks as Miss Idaho. So often I feel like I am alone: like I am the only person who has the "flaws" I have to live with, and everyone else is normal. Before Miss Idaho, I had only met a few other diabetics with type 1. I felt like one in a million, but in a bad way, with no one around who could understand me. The weeks following Miss Idaho changed that completely. I realized that there were millions of people (over 3 million in the U.S. alone, to be exact) who understood exactly what I was going through, because they were just like me: living with type 1! I wasn't weird or different. And I was no longer alone.

Throughout my year as Miss Idaho, I have spoken mainly at diabetes events, which are inevitably full of people living with diabetes. On the occasions that I have spoken at events that have nothing to do with diabetes, I usually end up briefly telling my story. The number of people who approach me afterwards and tell me that they also have diabetes or wear insulin pumps amazes me. I think we would all be surprised at how many people living with diabetes are around us without our even knowing or noticing them! I hope knowing that brings some peace to anyone who currently feels isolated with his or her disease, and I wish you could experience the overwhelming support that I did during the #showmeyourpump campaign. (If you need some encouragement, get on Instagram and check out the 5,000 people who have posted pump pictures, or get on Twitter to interact with the #DOC.) Thanks to the Diabetes Online Community I have been able to make connections from all over the world, and I hope that you can do the same.

8: My Miss Idaho Sugar Linings

The months after winning Miss Idaho were some of the most exciting, busy, and stressful months of my life. I was the very last Miss America contestant to be crowned, which meant that I had to turn in my paperwork extremely quickly. I also had only eight weeks to improve my talent, get a Miss America-worthy wardrobe, and continue to hone my interview skills, all while staying up-to-date on current events, and making time to eat healthy and go to the gym. It was insanity.

Add the results of #showmeyourpump on top of that, and you get…

… What the heck is crazier than insanity?

Anyways, I was beyond busy, but it was wonderful. Two years earlier, when I was diagnosed with diabetes, I thought nothing good would come out of it. Now, not only has some good come out of it, but being diagnosed with diabetes has become one of the most important things that has ever happened to me!

I've mentioned sugar linings before, and, of course, since that is the title of this book, you probably have an idea of what I mean by the term. You are most likely very familiar with the phrase "every cloud has a silver lining." For every unfortunate and negative event in our lives, there is something good that can come out of it. *Sugar lining* is my term for the blessings, benefits, and perks that come into our lives because of diabetes.

After Miss Idaho, my life was overwhelmed with sugar linings. Of course, there were the silly, trivial things, such as new Instagram and Twitter followers, as well as always finding my mailbox full of letters. These weren't life-changing things, but I definitely loved them!

Then, there were the more meaningful things. During the first few weeks after I posted the pump picture on Facebook, I had up to five interviews every day on the phone, over Skype, or sometimes even in person. That gave me the priceless opportunity to spread my message to hundreds of thousands of people who may have missed the Facebook post. I wanted the world to hear 1) that they should love the things that make them different, because these things make them unique; and 2) that life can throw awful things at us, but we can learn a lot from them, use them to become stronger as individuals, and let them inspire us to make a difference by serving those who are facing similar challenges. One of my favorite interviews resulted in an NPR article, written by Miriam Tucker (@MiriamETucker) that ended up being the #1 read NPR blog article for the year of 2014, receiving over 2.7 million hits! I was also featured on the Today Show, and Good Morning America came to my house in little Twin Falls, Idaho, to interview me. With all of the interviews and articles published, we estimate that my story reached well over 20 million people!

Most of my in-person interviews, as well as the Miss Idaho gym sponsor, and my pageant interview and walking coaches, were all located in Boise, which is about two hours away from where I live. I soon started staying with McCall and her family, which quickly resulted in our building an amazing friendship. She is only thirteen, and it was such a strange concept to me that one of my best friends didn't have a Facebook or a cellphone (not to mention that I had to constantly remind myself to keep boy-talk to a minimum). Nevertheless, I began spending the majority of my time with McCall and her brothers.

My life was an unbelievable whirlwind. I was flown down to Los Angeles for a health talk show, and soon after, I found myself on a plane to New York City after being invited to appear on the Dr. Oz Show. Since then, I have traveled all over the country after getting hired to speak at various events. It has been awesome. I definitely can't complain about being paid to travel and inspire others, but flying, staying in hotel rooms, and exploring foreign cities alone gets to be very lonely. Whenever people ask me what has been the greatest challenge during my year, I always respond that it has, hands down, been coping with loneliness. This New York trip was no different. I bought myself Broadway tickets for every evening I would be there, and spent the first couple of afternoons walking around Times Square by myself. It was fun, but every moment I still felt alone and wished I could share the experience with someone. Finally, the time came for me to be picked up and driven to the Dr. Oz Studio!

When the car pulled up to the studio, I was quickly ushered to my dressing room where I waited for about thirty minutes before being escorted to hair and make-up. Fifteen minutes after being escorted back to my dressing room, I left to wander the halls in search of a restroom. I was taken aback when everyone seemed flustered, and I realized I needed an escort in order to go anywhere, not just when I was shown the way to hair and make-up. I still didn't think much of it. It was different from other interviews and behind-the-scenes places I had been in before, but that was because Dr. Oz was a big deal. Higher security made sense, I guess. I was brought a binder with the script, full of the questions Dr. Oz would ask me so I could think about how I wanted to respond. There were some questions about my experience at Miss Idaho, about why I decided to wear my insulin pump, about my upcoming competition at Miss America, and, lastly, about how McCall had been impacted by my decision to wear my pump and what that meant to me.

Finally, it was time to go backstage. I was given a microphone, and some last minute make-up retouches. I then waited for the commercial break to end, and for Dr. Oz to call me on stage. Right as I heard my cue, the doors in front of me slid open automatically, music played, and the cameras swung to face me. It was unreal! I was in the most beautiful, high-end sound stage I had ever seen in my life. The studio audience cheered as pictures of the Miss Idaho competition, along with some other #showmeyourpump pictures from my Instagram followers, were displayed on the gigantic screens behind me. *It was so ridiculously cool*!

The interview went awesome. Dr. Oz was a lot of fun to talk to, and I was beyond excited to spread my message and diabetes awareness to the huge new audience he was helping me reach.

Before I knew it, the interview was over. He was asking me the last question. "Now, even though you haven't even worn your insulin pump at Miss America yet, you have already been able to witness first hand how your bravery in proudly wearing your pump has already made an impact on someone who is now very dear to your heart," he stated. "Tell me about the little girl who was backstage of Miss Idaho who was very touched by your decision to wear your medical device."

I proceeded to recount the events that had happened behind the scenes at Miss Idaho between McCall and me, as well as provide updates on what had happened since then, including the fact that McCall had nearly completed the process of getting her own insulin pump and was impatiently awaiting the day that her new t:slim would arrive.

"That's so wonderful!" Dr. Oz responded and sighed, "Wouldn't it be so fun if McCall was here in New York with you?"

Geez. He had no idea. As I am someone who gets pretty anxious in crowds, visiting Times Square alone wasn't as enjoyable as it could have been. Plus, McCall was one of my favorite people in the world, and I missed her like crazy.

Before I could respond, let alone realize what was happening, the automatic doors were opening again, while the welcome music replayed. I gasped. McCall was walking out! What?! Much like on the night I was crowned Miss Idaho, I don't remember much about what happened after that. Dr. Oz asked McCall a few questions, and we were whisked off the stage as our segment came to an end. All the while, I was attempting to comprehend what had just taken place!

I eventually managed to wrap my head around the fact that she was in New York—almost 2,500 miles away from where I had last seen her only forty-eight hours earlier! The rest of the day, I spent with McCall and her mom in Times Square shopping, catching a Broadway show, and, of course, treating ourselves to some New York cheesecake (accompanied by a great, big bolus of insulin). They filled me in on the lengths everyone went to in order to keep the surprise top secret: having me escorted to the bathroom, being booked at separate hotels, and even avoiding similar flight schedules, so we didn't accidentally run into each other during a layover. I couldn't believe it! It was one of the best surprises of my life, one of the highlights of my crazy, exciting year as Miss Idaho, and of course, a gigantic sugar lining!

When I was diagnosed with diabetes, my dad bought me loads of books on the topic, sent me links to articles about diabetes, and basically gave me any information he could possibly find about diabetes. He also bought me a subscription to Diabetes Forecast, produced by the America Diabetes Association (probably the most well known and most widely read diabetes magazine in the country). Throughout the many, many months between when I was diagnosed and when I won Miss Idaho, I was introduced to many celebrities with diabetes, whom I now list as my heroes, simply because they had the chance to appear on the cover of Diabetes Forecast. One of my favorite Miss Idaho sugar linings is the moment I received my October 2014 copy. I opened my mailbox, and pulled out the issue on which I had the honor of being featured on the cover. While I knew it was coming, it hadn't felt real until that day. Six months earlier, I would have never predicted how many amazing things would result from my diabetes diagnosis a couple years before.

• • •

At last, it was time to head to Miss America. I was actually going to wear my insulin pump on the Miss America stage in Atlantic City, New Jersey! If I were to write about my Miss America experience, I wouldn't even know where to start. Every moment during those two weeks was full of amazing sugar linings. There are fifty-two sugar linings from that week that I will remember for the rest of my life: the other young women who compete for Miss America are some of the most amazing, accomplished, intelligent, and compassionate people I have met. I will treasure their friendship forever!

For those of you who may not know me well, I have been a Miss America fanatic ever since I first heard about Nicole Johnson. Every year, I have followed the Pageant Junkies blog, trying to make my own predictions about who will win each state title. I also follow all fifty-three Miss America contestants on social media to choose my favorites, as well as make my predictions on who will win Miss America.

On the day of the Miss America competition, my Miss Idaho friends and I get together to watch. We call it our Super Bowl, and if you were there to witness us watching, you would understand. We often jump to our feet screaming when our favorite contestant advances or fall to the ground in agony when they get eliminated. It is crazy and emotional, but it makes for some of the best girls' nights of all time.

We also make a huge deal out of our predictions. At the beginning of the night, we each make a list of who we believe will make top

15, and which of those women will receive the People's Choice Award. Once the top 15 is revealed, we then make our guess as to who will advance to the top 12, and so on, through the top 10, top 5, the final placement, and the winner.

I'm fairly good at guessing because of how much I follow the women on social media. The way I usually predict the People's Choice Award, also referred to as America's Choice, is by checking out the YouTube views on each contestant's People's Choice video. The year before I won Miss Idaho, there were several contestants that I thought were really inspiring, and would be in the running. However, Teresa Vail, who ended up winning the award, killed the rest of the contestants in the number of times her video had been watched.

I knew that the best predictor of the People's Choice winner would be to watch the amount of views on everyone's videos. As the days passed by at Miss America, I was hoping to be the winner of that award. However, every night when we were allowed to check our phones, I would see that several states had many more views than my People's Choice video had during the week leading up to Miss America, and my heart sunk a little more each day. I also knew that only the women who made the top 15, including the People's Choice winner, get to compete on national television. But as the days in Atlantic City passed by, it was looking less and less likely that I would be one of them. There were thousands of kids living with type 1 who were going to watch Miss America that weekend, and were waiting to see me wearing my t:slim on nation television, and I couldn't let them down. I *had* to come up with a backup plan.

We started filming the introductions at the end of the first week. Each contestant had a chance to appear on television for a short amount of time at the beginning of the show. We had all come up with a cute little introduction that had something to do with the state we were representing. Since I was coming to the realization that the introduction was very possibly the only time I would be shown on TV, I decided to clip my t:slim Insulin Pump to the collar of my dress (a place I would never normally dream of wearing it) so that everyone could see it. "From the small town of Twin Falls, but representing diabetics worldwide," I exclaimed when my turn came, "I'm *your* little sweet potato, Miss Idaho, Sierra Sandison!" There. It was done. My insulin pump would definitely be shown on TV. I could relax now.

Competition week went by quickly. We interviewed at the beginning of the week and spent the following evenings competing. Before we knew it, finals night had arrived. I have been on stage a lot because my mom worked at a performing arts school for most of my life, but never had I ever felt as terrified as I did when the cameras starting rolling that evening. I thought I was going to be sick, and walking on stage was the last thing I wanted to do.

As we walked across the stage, through the audience, and down the catwalk, performing the opening number, I thought about all of the women that I had watched on TV in previous years. Many of them were heroes because of the message they had brought to the Miss America stage—the same stage I was now standing on. I reflected on how much I admired them: Nicole Kelley, Teresa Vail, Heather Whitestone, Claire Buffie, Allyn Rose, Mallory Hytes Hagan, Alexis Wineman, and of course, Nicole Johnson. They all had unique stories and had used them to diversify the Miss America stage, in addition to influencing those who had looked up to them, including myself. Now, after a lot of hard work and failure along the way, I was in the same position they had been in. I couldn't believe it was real.

Before I knew it, the opening number was over, and we were lining up to hear the name of the People's Choice winner before they read off of the names of fourteen other women who would also advance to the top 15. I glanced around, thinking about the other women who were just as, if not more, likely to advance as I was.

Miss Kentucky lives with Multiple Sclerosis, and we had bonded the past couple weeks over being "auto-immune-buddies"; Miss New Mexico had the support of 4-H groups nationwide, since that was her platform; Miss Alabama was a former Miss America's Outstanding Teen and a daughter of a former NFL player; Miss Mississippi had a huge social media following and had placed very well during her time on American Idol. Then there was the fact that, in the entire history of Miss America, Miss Idaho had only been a finalist once, forty-four years earlier at Miss America 1971. Who was I to think that this year would be different?

With all those thoughts racing through my head in the last few moments before Chris Harrison opened the envelope to read the name of the winner of America's Choice. "It was selfie palooza as each of our contestants posted a one-minute video on MissAmerica.org, Facebook, YouTube, and ABC.com. You logged on in record numbers, and made one contestant a semi-finalist. America's Choice may have also been a judges' choice." He read, as my heart began to sink. I was used to wanting something badly, such as the lead in a play, or a solo in choir, and always being let down. Why would this time be any different? Miss Idaho hadn't made the top 15 in 44 years! At least I was standing on the Miss America stage. That was a huge accomplishment in itself! Chris continued, "America, you chose...Miss Idaho, Sierra Sandison!" I was humbled and blown away when I realized it was *me*. Again, it was a blur. I only remember hearing "Idaho," which brought me to my knees in tears before I was ushered backstage to prepare for the swimsuit portion of the competition.

I, dorky *Sierra Sandison*, was actually going to compete at Miss America, on national television, *wearing my insulin pump*. More importantly, winning America's Choice meant more to me than the crown. Winning Miss America meant impressing seven judges; winning the People's Choice vote meant that I had touched lives and hearts nationwide. This is my greatest sugar lining to date.

In the months following Miss America, I spent the majority of my time traveling the country speaking about being proud of what makes us different, as well as using our obstacles and adversities to make us stronger, and to make a difference in the lives of others. I have been to over twenty states during my time as Miss Idaho and have traveled out-of-state almost every weekend throughout the year. It has been a dream come true. How many people get to travel *and* inspire others as their job?!

• • •

Finally, McCall has played a huge role in my story, and has been by my side through it all, so I thought it was only fitting to have her contribute to this book by sharing her side of the story in her own words:

"At the age of nine, I was diagnosed with type 1 diabetes on September 30th, 2011. I was terrified. I remember sitting in the doctor's office, I didn't understand anything he was saying. When my mom told me what was going on I burst into tears. My life had changed forever, and I was not happy about it. We went to the lab to get my blood drawn, and all I remember was screaming. I was terrified of the needle. When we got the results back, my blood sugar was 525. The doctor told us that we had to go into the diabetes center the next day, which really concerned my mom because my dad and brother were going out of town early the next morning, so she asked if we could wait until they got back a few days later. The doctor immediately responded very bluntly: "Absolutely not!" He told us that if we waited even one more day, I would be in the ICU, most likely in a coma.

"The next day, Friday, my mom and I got into the car and drove to our 10:45am appointment at the Humphrey's Diabetes Center in Boise, Idaho. I remember my mind just racing as I got out of the car. I had no idea what was about to happen. We sat down in the office and waited for the nurse to come in and start explaining what we would have to do every day for the rest of my life. As she explained I tried to listen, but I had a million questions racing through my head: "Can I still play sports?" "Can I still do everything I'm doing now?" "Can I still eat candy?" All of those fears were calmed a bit when she reassured me that I could live a normal life with this new disease. But I still had one more question: "Why me?" The nurse didn't have an answer, and that's when I started to become angry. She then showed me how to check my blood and told me what insulin was. And then the scariest part of all: the first shot. My mom gave me my first shot and all my shots after that for one month. As we left the diabetes center, I didn't say a word. I was furious. I remember sitting in the car with my blanket over my head crying the whole time. I didn't talk to anyone but myself, and I just kept asking myself, "Why me? Why me?!?!" over and over. I then turned to the Lord. I prayed and asked him, and soon after, I came across the quote "You were given this life because you are strong enough to live it." After that, I knew that everything happened for a reason and the Lord had a plan for me.

"When I was first diagnosed, I wanted nothing to do with my diabetes. I especially didn't want to talk about two things in particular: getting an insulin pump, and going to diabetes camp! The pump would make my disease visible, and I didn't want to go to camp and talk about the thing I hated most: my diabetes. After about two years, my doctor finally convinced me to go to camp. I loved it! I went to Camp Hodia for a whole week, and I had the time of my life! I met so many great friends and I learned things about diabetes that I didn't even know. I even gave myself a shot in my arm for the first time! Camp was also filled with crafts, games, swimming, horseback riding, a carnival, cabin skits, a trip to Sun Valley, and some pretty delicious meals. It was definitely an experience I will never forget!

"After camp, my parents picked me up, and my mom had some exciting news! She was Mrs. Idaho 2007, and ever since then I had wanted to be just like her. You have to be at least 13 to compete in Miss Idaho's Outstanding Teen, and for years I had been counting down the days until I was old enough! I still had a while, but my mom was excited to tell me that she had just found out there would be a Miss Idaho's Outstanding Preteen pageant starting that fall. I was ecstatic!

"I began preparing for the Miss Idaho's Outstanding Preteen Pageant. I practiced interview and talent, and I even found the perfect evening gown! When October finally rolled around, I competed against five other beautiful young ladies in the categories of private interview, talent, fitness, evening gown, and onstage question, and…I won! I was crowned Miss Idaho's Outstanding Preteen 2014! I was very excited, but I had no idea that just a few months later, my life would change even more. After my crowning I had so much fun making appearances with my sister queens Heidi Olsen, Miss Idaho's Outstanding Teen 2014, and Sarah Downs, Miss Idaho 2013. We can only hold a title for one year and that meant that when the Miss Idaho pageant happened in July, Sarah would have to give up her crown.

"July finally came, and it was time to crown a new Miss Idaho! The Miss Idaho Pageant is two nights long: preliminaries and finals. On the night of prelims, I was standing backstage and I saw that one of the contestants was wearing what I thought was an insulin pump so I walked up to her and asked her if it was an insulin pump. She seemed a bit flustered by my question, and I knew how she felt: I hated getting questions from strangers about my diabetes. I quickly reassured her by telling her that I was also diabetic, and that I had always been afraid to get a pump because I thought that I would get made fun of by my peers at school. This contestant was, of course, the one and only, Sierra Sandison! I didn't know this at the time, but Sierra later told me that she went out onstage not caring if she won or not, she just wanted to show me that I was beautiful, insulin pump and all. At the end of that first night, I had made the decision to get an insulin pump. Sierra was so happy and she said that no matter what happened on finals night, she had worn her pump for me. My mom was in tears talking to

Sierra, but she also didn't think we would be able to afford the pump, and hoped she could find a way. The next night, Sierra was crowned Miss Idaho 2014!

"In August I received some exciting news: I was asked to surprise Sierra on the Dr. Oz show! I was very excited! I was able to fly to New York City with my mom and explore everything for three days. We went to two Broadway shows and did almost every other tourist thing imaginable. Meeting Dr. Oz was pretty cool, too! When it came time to leave I was very sad, but I had such a great time, and I had something to look forward to when I got home. I had been counting down the days. I could not wait! Finally, the day came. The day I had been waiting for: the day I got my t:slim Pump!

"I was thrilled! I was going back to the same place, and same office that I had been to the day after my diagnosis, but this time I was much happier! I remember that I was not able to sit still because I was so excited! When the nurse finally came in, she started telling us lots of information about the pump and lots of things we needed to know about it! I was not able to insert the infusion set at first because I was kind of scared, but after a few weeks, I was finally able to do it on my own. To this day, I am completely self-reliant! I can check my own blood sugar, count my own carbs, deliver my own insulin and work my pump all by myself!

I am very proud of myself, seeing how far I've come since that first day. I am so thankful for everyone who has helped me since I was diagnosed, but I think this year has been the best! Over the last year and a half, my life has changed more than I could have ever imagined...all because of one very special princess, and her pump."

Of course, one of the most meaningful sugar linings that happened because of Miss Idaho has been doing for others what Nicole Johnson once did for me. Now that I am home from Miss America, it never fails to put a smile on my face when I bring McCall lunch at school and see her come running across the cafeteria to greet me...with her insulin pump clipped to the collar of her sweatshirt, where I put it during my Miss America introduction. Being able to form a friendship with McCall, and see her beam with confidence in her diabetes has meant the world to me.

· · ·

I often find myself reflecting back on my first few months of living with diabetes. Every day I would remind myself how unfair it was that I, out of all of my relatives with a genetic predisposition for the disease, was the one who had to live with it. Why me? I didn't take care of myself at all throughout this period. I constantly felt sick because of all the extreme highs and lows that my indifference was causing me. I even quit the track team that spring because of the physical whirlwind I was caught in. I looked back at the day I was diagnosed, February 12th, 2012, and thought of it as the worst day of my life.

That day was a sad, traumatic, and devastating day. There is nothing fun about being told that you have a disease that will require you to poke yourself with many needles, all day, every day, for the rest of your life. What is even worse is finding out that there is no cure. However, while the day I was diagnosed isn't necessarily a pleasant memory in my mind, I have since realized that being diagnosed with diabetes was one of the most important things that could have ever happened to me.

9: The Cloud

I know what you are probably thinking at this point: "*of course* diabetes was the best thing that ever happened to *her*! She became Miss Idaho. However, the chances of me/my child ever doing something like going to Miss America are pretty slim."

The previous chapters were primarily dedicated to the sugar linings that came into my life thanks to my involvement in the Miss America Organization. They have been huge blessings and *very* exciting. However, I would have to say that some of my favorite, most priceless, and most important sugar linings are not related to becoming Miss Idaho at all. In fact, they are sugar linings that every single one of us who live with type 1 may have at some point, and when they come into your life, I hope you recognize them as sugar linings too.

The truth is, diabetes isn't awesome. It sucks most of the time! We all know that.

While diabetes can't stop us from doing anything—whether that is competing at Miss America, going to the Olympics, studying abroad, going to slumber parties, or maybe just playing a sport in high school—it makes all of those things slightly, if not a lot, more difficult. We have to be constantly worried about our safety and health: What's my blood sugar right now? And will this activity affect it? If there's an emergency, do I have access to treatment? If I'm out of town, or out of the country, and my insulin gets overheated or I break the vial, will I be able to replace it quickly enough? There is a constant cloud of worry looming over us that people with functioning pancreases don't have to deal with.

This chapter is about the cloud, and sometimes the storm, that constantly looms over us: the negative side of diabetes and how we deal with it. I hate thinking and talking about the clouds in my life, tending instead to focus mostly on the positive. However, I know that at some points during my disease, my diabetes cloud has done a very great job at hiding the sugar linings that lie behind it. Recently, it has been the opposite: I have forced my cloud to hide behind my huge sugar linings, which in turn has caused me to run into a bit of writer's block for this chapter. To help me, I decided to reach out to my twitter followers and ask them: What is the most difficult thing for you about living with diabetes?

I was surprised by some of the answers, but I shouldn't have been! I am still on my parents insurance, and they make sure they never let me feel guilty about the huge financial burden my diabetes creates. I was surprised, then, to see this as one of the most common responses to my question! Several young adults expressed that dealing with the financial aspect was a huge deal for them. I am very blessed for now, but I definitely need to work my diabetes expenses into my future budget.

Dealing with the misinformed comments that people make can be extremely emotionally draining, as well. I recently posted a video to Facebook called "*What NOT to say to a parent of a type 1 diabetic*". It could also be called *What NOT to say to ANY person with type 1 diabetes* (and of course family members of T1Ds). Most of us are very familiar with the items on the list of things you shouldn't say and can likely predict what's on it. I encourage you to watch the video, however, because the robot voices it uses are fairly similar to the monotone, sassy comebacks to misinformed commenters that are constantly flying through my head (and probably yours as well). Plus, it's freaking hilarious. Make sure to look it up!

Speaking of parents of type 1 diabetics, shout out to you! I recently returned home from a mother-daughter conference. At certain points during the conference, the mothers and daughters would be separated for different sessions and seminars. I would always be with the daughters, and at one specific point we were running around the room, playing icebreakers, jumping in and out of a rented photo booth, and having a blast with our new DiaBuddies. One of the girls, who had attended the conference previously, laughed about how much fun we were having, but then said, "How much you wanna bet the moms are in the other room crying?" Sure enough, I had to go into the other conference room to grab something, and the moms were hysterical. We had a laugh about it back in the teen room, but it once again reminded me of what I've always felt to be true: it might actually be more stressful being a parent of a child with type 1, than being a diabetic. Parents of kids with T1D are…well, I don't even have an adjective to describe them, but I have so much respect for them. I can't imagine how heartbroken and worried I would be if I knew my child had a chronic disease that I had no power to take away from them.

These parents experience sleepless nights due to late-night blood sugar checks, and long days at work worrying about whether or not the teachers and school nurse will know how to treat the inevitable highs and lows. You wait for a text from a teen at a slumber party to make sure they are okay, and anxiously watch a high school basketball game while paying more attention to the numbers on your Dexcom SHARE app than the ones on the scoreboard.

One mom tweeted me and said that the most difficult part of parenting a type 1 teen was trying to balance her concern for their health, while still allowing her teen to be independent and pursue opportunities that can seem risky for a diabetic. I could relate to that, especially, because of the preparation that led up to my trips to Cambodia and Europe. Parents can often be torn between protecting their teen/emerging adult, while still wanting to encourage them to believe that type 1 diabetes can't hold them back from achieving their dreams and living a normal life. If I were a parent, I would imagine that dealing with such a huge contradiction would be one of the greatest challenges I would have to face.

On my journey, one of the worst aspects of having diabetes is not being allowed to take a break from life when my blood sugars aren't cooperating. As a public speaker, when I am flown across the country to a conference and wake up in my hotel the day of my speech feeling awful, I can't just "call into work sick." I'm sure we all feel this way sometimes. We wish our blood sugars were less stubborn on the days we feel we need to stay in bed all day, instead of going to school or work. One [exhausting] week, I had a schedule packed full of school appearances. When I visit schools, I get in contact with the local diabetes community and give an assembly at each school with a type 1 student. After telling my story, I explain the basics of diabetes, and refute common misconceptions in the hope of eliminating any bullying based on diabetes. This particular week, my insulin had gotten overheated and it took me three days to realize that it wasn't a pump problem. Since I was out of state, it was impossible to reschedule the schools assemblies. I knew that calling and telling the kids that Miss Idaho was cancelling the appearance at their school wasn't an option. I had had an incident earlier when I was scheduled to speak at Avery A.'s school—she and her mom, Hallie, are behind The Princess and the Pump blog. When the speech was cancelled due to a bomb threat, Avery was beyond devastated. I felt so powerless. I never wanted to see a child that disappointed again. I especially didn't want it to happen if *I* was the one making the decision to cancel, so I stuck it out. The entire week, I was exhausted, but I didn't quit. Either way, I still feel guilty every time I have to work with miserable blood sugars. I always hope to make an impact on everyone in the audience, and if my energy is low and focus is off, I can't do my best. I hate my diabetes for the times it has caused me to feel like I let people down when my speeches haven't been as great as they should have been because of my blood sugars. The most frustrating part of the cloud for me is that diabetes can often make me feel like a failure.

I empathized with all of the responses I received, but one really resonated with my personal experience. "Those really bad days," @JSchwenken tweeted, "when it seems everything you've done to be successful, fails." It's discouraging to know that even if I focused 100% of my energy checking my blood sugar constantly and always bolusing the perfect amount at the perfect time, I would still have out-of-range blood sugars on occasion! As I said earlier, I don't like spending energy on activities I know I will "fail" at. Recently, while in the Bay Area, the wonderful Katie Craft (an awesome T1D that I hope you all have the good fortune of meeting someday) mentioned the language they are careful to use in her family, as well as the diabetes camp she grew up at, in order to avoid the feeling of failure. Instead of asking someone to "please test" his or her blood sugar, they say, "Please check". The word "test" implies that it is something the diabetic will either pass or fail, and as Moira McCarthy says, the numbers are simply information. Any information is good information. After the teen or child checks—no matter what the number is—the parent (or camp counselor) replies, "thank you for checking", rather than getting angry and reacting to the child having a "bad" number. Remember: there is no such thing as bad information or a bad number. Understanding that concept has helped prevent me from kicking myself when I see a big yellow mountain stretch across my Dexcom screen, and to not get discouraged or give up because of the days my blood sugar decides it hates me a little extra than usual.

. . .

When I walked into my Miss Idaho interview, the very first question the judges asked me was, "What is the most difficult thing about living with diabetes?" I thought about it for a few seconds. I try to focus on the positive, so I had never given it much thought. Since getting my Dexcom and pump, I experienced enough freedom and control that I hadn't suffered much from burnout recently. I was at a point where I had accepted that having "bad" blood sugars was just a part of living with diabetes, and forgave myself, especially when I knew I was trying my absolute best and out-of-range numbers were simply caused by my body being mean and unpredictable. It was still awful. Constantly dealing with highs and lows was the obvious choice for "the most difficult thing," but I felt like there was something deeper hurting me than having to regulate a certain part of my digestive system. While I had suffered physically, I knew the thing that hurt the worst was something psychological and emotional. Was it the constant stress that came along with worrying about my blood sugar? No. The fear of having complications in the future? No. Those could definitely be the greatest burdens for many of you. The more people I meet with type 1 diabetes, the more I believe that the greatest struggles that come with this disease are rarely physical. What's the hardest part for you? It could be fear. It could be loneliness. It could be frustration. It could be the never-ending feeling of failure. The most difficult thing about diabetes is almost always emotional.

I knew what mine was, but I was embarrassed to admit it. I couldn't come up with a different answer, so I decided to be honest. "I know it may seem silly, but I was diagnosed when I was already a self-conscious, dorky teenage girl, and had already bullied in middle school and parts of high school. Honestly, the most difficult thing about diabetes for me has been coming to terms with being different," I confessed, "Having my peers know that I had diabetes—a disease that has a negative connotation already, is the butt of too many jokes, and is commonly misunderstood—was difficult enough. Add in the scars from shots and sites, not to mention having to be attached to medical devices in the first place, and diabetes is a teenage girl's worst nightmare! Dealing with the body image issues that adolescents face is hard enough without diabetes. The greatest challenge I have faced with diabetes is learning to love myself and be confident while living with it."

At the time, I thought I was being ridiculous and shallow. I was living with a life-threatening disease, and I just told the judges that the most difficult thing about it was worrying ABOUT HOW I LOOKED? "You shouldn't have been that honest," I told myself, "Geez. Shallow much, Sierra?"

Shallow, no. Human, yes. A few days later, I discovered that I wasn't the only one who felt this way. As letters, pictures, and stories poured in as a result of the #showmeyourpump campaign, I realized that struggling with body image was common among diabetics—*very* common. Even more surprising, it wasn't just a teenage girl problem! Men, women, girls, and boys of all ages were letting me know that one of their greatest challenges of living with diabetes was trying not be ashamed of their bodies. I heard how my decision to wear my insulin pump inspired them and gave them a much needed confidence boost. Even for those that weren't necessarily struggling with body image issues, it seemed common that the emotional burdens often outweighed the physical ones.

Diabetes freaking sucks, for an endless list of reasons! I don't need to tell you that. What I do want to tell you is that there is a bright side to living with type 1 diabetes or whatever difficult situation you may be facing in your life. The sugar linings you find may or may not outweigh the cloud that looms over you, but they are still worth looking for. I hope I can help you find them.

10: Strength

Wow. The previous chapter was exhausting to write. Thank goodness I'm not writing an entire book on clouds! Let's get back to the awesome stuff: sugar linings. What could possibly make every struggle that I just vented about tolerable? For me, and most diabetics that I have been able to meet during my travels, there are quite a few things!

Diabetes has made me stronger. As most adversities do, it has taught me that I can handle more than I ever imagined I could. I am proud of the discipline it requires to maintain my blood sugars all day, every day, and I have been able to apply that dedication and work ethic to other areas of my life.

It has brought me friends (fellow diabetics) who are going through the same struggles as I am. Their friendships are priceless, especially since they understand what I am going through at a deeper level than anyone else does. Those who have lived with diabetes longer than I have are my inspirations. It is so encouraging to have relationships with people who are living healthy and amazing lives with this disease, and knowing that they have done it for ten, thirty, fifty years, or more years helps me get through the days when I want to give up.

Living with diabetes has given me a passion and purpose: serving the diabetes community. I have been able to make a difference, which is something I would never, ever trade—even if it meant going back in time and somehow erasing my experience with diabetes.

Finally, having had to struggle with diabetes has been difficult, but it's even more difficult when others don't understand. When uneducated people assume that I caused my disease by living an unhealthy lifestyle, and judge me, it hurts! It's unbelievably frustrating when someone gets mad about my being late due to my not being able to drive because of a low. Diabetes, along with other adversities I face in my life, has taught me to never judge others who are different from me or make assumptions about them. I try my best to empathize with them and put myself in their shoes. I may not completely understand them or know what they are going through, but I try my best to comprehend how they must feel. Because of my experience with diabetes, I hope to never be the person who causes someone pain from unnecessary judgment.

Diabetes has given me a greater ability to show compassion and empathy.

Strength, friendships, opportunities to serve others, and increased compassion and empathy are the sugar linings that diabetes has brought into my life that I wouldn't trade for the world. However, I didn't realize them immediately. In fact, it was my fellow diabetics who helped me discover them by sharing their own stories of struggles and joy (yes, joy!) that come along with living with type 1. I hope to discover more as my journey with diabetes continues, and in the meantime, hope I can be an encouragement to you, just as my "DiaBesties" have been to me by sharing the sugar linings that we can all find if we are willing to look for them.

• • •

How many times have we heard, "what doesn't kill you makes you stronger"? (Thank you Kelly Clarkson.) Or, as Friedrich Nietzsche, a nineteenth-century German philosopher with a crazy name, once said, "that which does not destroy us, makes us stronger."

(But seriously Nietzsche, I didn't know you were even allowed to have five consonant letters in a row. Goodness gracious!)

That statement, along with those pop song lyrics, is repeated over and over again because of the truth it holds. The adversities we face in our lives make us stronger. This is true both emotionally *and* physically.

When we go to the gym and lift weights, it's not a particularly pleasant feeling. We are literally breaking down our existing muscle. Over the course of the next few days, the muscle rebuilds itself and becomes stronger. As my gym rat friends like to say: no pain, no gain. The same is true for "emotional" gains—however, *that* pain is usually a lot more difficult to bear than the burn in your glutes while doing a squat.

Diabetes has shown me what I'm capable of. Things I didn't even know I could do without my disease, such as backpacking alone through Europe for five months, I have successfully done with diabetes on board! In fact, it makes it an even greater accomplishment knowing that I not only did something that the average person would find scary, but I did it with an extra obstacle in my way.

I like to tell kids that we stick needles in our body constantly— something that the rest of the world is terrified of! If we are brave enough to deal with that, along with everything else that comes along with diabetes, we are brave enough to do anything. Diabetes is not an easy thing to deal with, but having to live with it makes us stronger, braver, and better prepared to deal with difficult circumstances that may arise in our futures.

11: DiaBesties

I grew up and was diagnosed in the small Idaho town of Twin Falls. It's actually considered one of the "major cities" in Idaho, but its population is a mere 45,981 (according to Google on the day I am writing this) so...I'll let you form your own opinion on how big or small you think Twin Falls is. In Idaho, at the time of this writing, we don't have our own Juvenile Diabetes Research Foundation (JDRF) or American Diabetes Association (ADA) chapters, and instead are adopted by the chapters in our neighboring states (Utah, Montana, Oregon, and Washington).

Today, I am extremely privileged to travel out of state almost every weekend in order to speak at various diabetes conferences, retreats, and camps. I make appearances at diabetes support groups, and sometimes stay with the families I have grown close to. I have met many influential diabetics that I follow on social media or by blog, such as Moira McCarthy, the author of *Raising Teens with Diabetes*; Sean Busby, a professional backcountry snowboarder who founded Riding on Insulin, all while living with T1D; Ryan Reed, a professional NASCAR driver with T1D; the wonderful Addington ladies from The Princess and the Pump blog; Kyle Cochran, and America Ninja Warrior (and his diabetes alert dog, Leeloo); Kerri Sparling, author of *Balancing Diabetes*, and blogger of SixUntilMe.com; and, of course, Nicole Johnson, and many, many more! I have had the pleasure to meet Derek Rapp, the CEO of JDRF. I have crossed paths with Jeff Hitchcock, who started Friends for Life, and hosts the well-known Children with Diabetes conference in Orlando every summer (which I can't wait to attend for the first time this year)! And in addition to the "DiaCelebs" that I meet regularly, I am constantly surrounded with other amazing people who either live with diabetes or have a loved one with diabetes.

I am surrounded by people with diabetes. I love it. I didn't realize how accustomed to it I had become until a few weeks ago. My boyfriend was running a half marathon he had been training for, and I had the weekend off, so I went to watch the race start (and later wait at the finish line with some friends). While we were in line at the registration table, a man walked by with a Dexcom on his arm. I didn't even look twice. Then, ten seconds after the man had disappeared into the crowd I freaked out! THAT GUY HAD DIABETES! We aren't even at a "diabetic gathering"! OH-EMM-FREAKING-GEE!

All of a sudden, I remembered that feeling. I had had it before.
Living in Twin Falls, there were no support groups or any kind of
diabetes chapters for me to participate in and meet other people
like myself. I was alone. There was a boy in high school a year
behind me who had type 1, as well as a girl I later met in college (I
love you, Colby and Maddie). I didn't know anyone else my age
with diabetes for a long time, but on a rare occasion that I saw
someone else with an insulin pump, whether I saw someone across
the produce section at the grocery store or a child in a park wearing
a Dexcom site, it made me feel better! Many people are fortunate
to live in an area with amazing diabetes organizations that are
supportive and encouraging—two of my favorites are ConnecT1D
in Seattle and CarbDM in the Bay Area. However, most of you may
be like me when I was first diagnosed: in a smaller area with no, or
very few, local resources. I spent the first three days after I was
diagnosed crying in my bedroom. I finally came out after having
gone online and discovered the DOC (Diabetes Online
Community). They were on Instagram sharing funny diabetes
memes and on Twitter venting about their blood sugar struggles.
There were endless diabetes Facebook groups for every
demographic I could think of. The emotions they shared through
their blogs resonated deeply with me and often brought me to
tears, but they were also strangely comforting. I wasn't alone.

People had felt like this before. They had experienced what I was now facing. More importantly, they're alive and well. It gave me hope: if they could do it, maybe I could too.

Recently, Kim Vlasnik, the blogger behind TextingMyPancreas.com and founder of the You Can Do This Project, posted a video of a speech she gave about diabetes (watch it here).

"For me, the hard part isn't the physical pain of finger sticks or injections, or the skin that rips off along with the adhesive of the medical devices I wear," she admits. "The hard part isn't even managing the fluctuating blood sugars or trying to manage and interpret all of the data I collect about myself each day. The hard part isn't even the long drawn out battles with insurance companies to gain the privilege of using the medical devices that can help keep me healthy and productive." She goes on to explain that the hard part for her is the psychosocial impact: "the cognitive burden of trying to manage a disease so insidious and pervasive, and never getting a break from it". She continues on, saying that the hard part is dealing with the fear of developing complications later in life, as well as how diabetes affects how she feels about herself and her body image. How difficult it is to do everything right and still not get the results she wants. These, along with the other emotional issues she lists, are things we are all too familiar with. Finally, she says how difficult it was to feel alone and to fight off the urge to commit self-harm. "What I didn't know then is how crucial to my health it would be to hear two small words: me too," Kim says, before explaining how it felt to finally find a community of other people living with diabetes—a community that knew what she was feeling. Instead of isolated, she felt empowered.

Me too. Those words make everything seem so much more tolerable. My heroes are the people living with diabetes who, just by example, show me that I can't give up just because of one day full of uncooperative blood sugars. They understand me. They are reassurance that I am not alone in my battle.

My diagnosis, unfortunately, came too late for me to ever attend diabetes camp as a camper. I have heard nothing but great things about camp! It allows the parents to take a break from the constant worry that accompanies diabetes, and it also gives the campers a chance to feel normal. When everyone else around you is checking their blood sugar, wearing pumps, and pulling out needles (that would, in most circumstances, be fairly conspicuous), you no longer have to feel different, weird, or that something is wrong with you. I may never have gotten to go to diabetes camp, but I know how amazing that feeling is from my involvement and experience with diabetes organizations across the country! It's an incredible and relieving feeling to have the people who surround you understand exactly what you're going through.

As I said in an earlier chapter, the most amazing experience I have had with the DOC was during the weeks that followed the launch of the #showmeyourpump campaign. Since I only knew a few diabetics in person, I felt pretty alone. All of us, whether or not we are living with diabetes, feel alone at times. For me, having to test my blood sugar, give myself shots, and wear an insulin pump made me feel weird. I felt like the only one in 7 billion that had to live like this. All of a sudden, thousands of people started sending me pictures, along with their stories of living with diabetes. For the first time, I felt as if having diabetes was almost…normal. There weren't just ten other people like me, or a hundred, or a thousand. I wasn't actually that weird or different after all! With over 3 million people in the U.S. alone who live with T1D, that means there are sixty times more people living with type 1 diabetes in our country than the entire population of my hometown! Mind=blown.

I have since had the opportunity to travel to and be involved with a lot of the country's most amazing diabetes organizations (one of which may have been in *your* city)! I have met many fellow diabetics and formed priceless friendships that I will cherish the rest of my life. McCall is an obvious example, and luckily, she's right here in Idaho with me all the time! She has become like a little sister to me, and I don't know what I would do without her sometimes. Another one of my closest DiaBesties is Hadley George from Cincinnati, Ohio.

Hadley is, first and foremost, one of the most impressive and articulate 16-year-olds I have ever met. And actually, she is probably one of the most impressive and articulate people of any age that I know!

Based on my first impression, emailing back and forth with her in the weeks leading up to my first Cincinnati event, I thought she was a [very professional] 35-year-old woman who held a position, such as program coordinator or event manager, for the organization that invited me—Type One Teens. They were throwing a huge gala for teens living with type 1, in honor of Diabetes Awareness Month, and also had smaller events once a month to give local teenagers with diabetes the opportunity to network with each other (a.k.a., hang out and talk about diabetes or, as most of us teens with T1D prefer, talk about anything *but* diabetes for once). These are my favorite diabetes organizations to work with: ones that give us the chance to meet other diabetics for support, or just the chance to feel normal and have other people surrounding us who understand.

I show up at the Cincinnati airport and am greeted by a small high school girl, holding a sign that says "Welcome Miss Idaho!" along with a bag of Chick-fil-A chicken nuggets—my favorite. Whoever this girl was, I loved her (and Cincinnati) already. "Maybe this is Mrs. George's daughter," I thought to myself, assuming that Hadley was waiting outside in the car. But, as you probably guessed, the small 16-year-old waiting for me at the baggage claim was Hadley herself.

We had the time of our lives that week: running around her house with her younger sisters, singing Frozen songs at the top of our lungs, eating lots of Chick-fil-A and grilled cheese sandwiches (another one of my favorites), and finally, attending the Believe In Blue gala at the end of the week. At some point during my visit, I had learned that Hadley was the founder, as well as the one mostly in charge, of the Type One Teens organization. I was extra impressed by the beautiful event she hosted, complete with an incredible turnout, venue, dancing, and generous sponsors. More importantly, she has created a huge network for Ohio teens living with T1D to thrive in all year-round!

Since my first visit to Cincinnati, Hadley and I remain in close contact. I also had the chance to go back to Ohio for another event and spent almost two weeks with the George family. We rant about the Bachelor together (well…at the time of this writing we are now just counting down the days until the next Bachelorette season premieres—#teamkaitlyn), are constantly on each others top snap chat friends' list, have gotten hooked on each other's favorite TV shows, and blast Taylor Swift on every car ride we share together. More importantly, she's been there to cry with me when my blood sugar refuses to come down. We have vented to each other when feeling depressed about how it sometimes seems that diabetes defines us and our lives—with me being primarily known as the "diabetic beauty queen", and her spending most of her free time running Type One Teens. It's always comforting being around someone else whose car is full of fruit snacks, and whose mom keeps the fridge filled with juice boxes. She gets me in a way my friends without diabetes do not. And, as I said in my dedication, her friendship is priceless and "is worth every finger poke, every bolus, every bad-blood-sugar-sick feeling, and every site change I will ever have to complete in my life." I am so grateful for Hadley, and all the other amazing friends I have met who also live with diabetes.

I asked Hadley to share a little bit about why she started Type One Teens.

Thanks for contributing, Hads!

"One super stormy scary night in December, in the middle of my diabetes burnout, I had essentially given up. The only way I thought I could make my diabetes go away was by ignoring it.

"While sitting in bed that evening, all I wanted was to talk to someone who had diabetes and knew what I was going through. I only knew a couple of people with type one, but I wasn't close to any of them. I needed a friend who could comprehend what it felt like to have a high or low blood sugar, or who knew how annoying it can be to change a pump set, along with the other struggles that come along with diabetes. Once I set my mind to something, I don't stop until I have accomplished it: I had to create a way to make friends with other teenagers who also lived with type one diabetes.

"The only logical conclusion I had was to create some sort of environment where teens with diabetes could come, have fun, and get to know one another. I knew no normal teenager would ever want to attend an event in order to talk about anything related to his or her diabetes. Therefore I needed a social group—not a support group: a place where teens could hang out, form friendships with people who face similar challenges, and most importantly, have fun!

"Teenagers would never want to sit in a circle and share their feelings. I needed to create an environment that was fun, yet supportive at the same time.   Type One Teens meets monthly at

various fun, social locations in the Greater Cincinnati area. We do not talk about diabetes, nor do we try to instill change in people— we simply hang out! On the occasion that diabetes is brought up, we are in a safe environment in which everyone knows exactly how the others feel—no nagging, no scolding, but instead, empathy and understanding. Type One Teens is a social group created by teens, for teens that provides exactly what every teenager struggling with type one diabetes needs: advice, support, and friendship from someone their same age who understands what they're going through.

"The monthly meetings are a blast, the attendance is amazing, and we always have such a wonderful time. But after a while, it wasn't enough for me. I wanted to spread awareness for teenagers who face the challenges of living with type one diabetes. I wanted a way for the peers of teens who have type one diabetes to be more informed about the disease in order to better support their friend when the person with T1D is both away from their parents and away their friends from Type One Teens. So, did I throw a seminar to better educate the general teenage population on what diabetes was? No! It had to be fun.

"The best way to do this was to have a dance. Most teenagers love to dress up and go to school dances. In my mind, I imagined a Gala for teenagers: disguising "diabetes education" (zzzzzzzzzzzzzz) as a fun night of dancing and glamor!

"The event is now known as "Believe in Blue." It is held in November (Diabetes Awareness Month) and is named after the official diabetes awareness color: blue. I chose "Believe in Blue" because we have something to believe in: if we believe that we can make living with this disease better, there will be a change.

"At Believe in Blue there was a vendor fair. This served as a perfect opportunity for teenagers with type one to see the latest technology in the diabetes world—I even heard that a few people who attended ended up making the decision to get an insulin pump after the event! The night was filled with fun: a DJ, photo booth, food and awesome diabetes related raffle prizes! However, the best part of the night was our special guest who we invited to speak during dinner to inform us about diabetes, as well as share her message to everyone of using our adversities to make us stronger: Sierra Sandison, Miss Idaho 2014—also known as my new best friend.

"I will let Sierra take over from here, but remember to HOPE. There will always be ups and downs, but stay strong and don't let diabetes win."

Hadley has been able to touch the lives of so many Cincinnati teens that also live with type one! The feeling of being surrounded by others who are just like you is incredible.

To anyone who feels alone: I promise, you are not! If you haven't already, I encourage you to get involved in the DOC and if possible, your local diabetes community. The friendships and connections you will form are priceless and will keep you going at the lowest points of your journey. Finally, thank you to everyone I have met during my own diabetes experience! You all mean the world to me, and I could never have gotten to where I am today without your support. Having you in my life is a much-needed reminder that I am not the only one.

12: Finding Our Passion. Making A Difference.

When I speak at schools, there is one part of my speech that I absolutely love. "Who wants to change the world during their life?" I always ask. "Who wants to make a difference before they die?" All of their hands instantly shoot up—right along with my goose bumps. Being an optimist, I like to think that most humans have a natural desire to do something important and improve the lives of others. I guess a pessimist might agree by saying that they do too, but only to ensure they leave a legacy behind. Either way, I think in general, we all enjoy the rewards of giving back and serving those around us.

One of the topics I often speak about is using the obstacles we face in life and turning them into opportunities. Many of those opportunities we have already discussed in this book: they give us a chance to shape ourselves and grow stronger as individuals. Adversity offers an opportunity to bond with people facing the same challenges that we do. Finally, difficult circumstances can show us where our passion lies. "Making a difference" is a broad statement, and while growing up (before we discover ourselves and our identities), we struggle with trying to decide exactly *how* we want to change the world. Facing a challenge life throws at us can sometimes give us the answer.

Veterans, as well as people with family members in the military, work hard to show our troops gratitude and support other military families. People who have had family members suffer from homelessness or have been homeless themselves will often feel compelled to give back to the local homeless shelter. When you participate in a JDRF walk or other fundraiser, most of the other attendees will also have a connection to T1D. This isn't always true, but often when volunteering with an organization, most of the people involved have some personal experience with the cause that inspired them to be there.

If the suffering we endure can give us a passion for something, or help us figure out how we want to make a difference with our lives, that is an amazing sugar lining! Volunteering, advocacy, and service are incredibly rewarding. And, who better to serve the diabetes community and offer advice on dealing with the disease than someone who has dealt with type 1 diabetes themselves?

One of the reasons I admire Hadley George so much is that she has not only used her experience with diabetes to become a stronger person, but she has also taken her disease and found a way to use it to touch the lives of others who are experiencing the same things she is. She recognized a way to help other teens who felt as alone as she did by taking the initiative to make Type One Teens a reality!

However, as I mentioned earlier, as much as Hadley and I enjoy giving back to the diabetes community, we sometimes feel as if we let diabetes define us. Of course, this isn't true all the time. In fact, the majority of the time, we are proud of the way we use our adversity as a reason to make a difference. I definitely loved meeting hundreds of people at various diabetes conferences this year and hopefully have made an impact on their lives by sharing my story. But I would be lying if I told you there aren't times at which I just want to escape the label of "diabetic", ignore the fact that I live with diabetes, and walk into a room and be greeted by "Hi Sierra!" rather than "Hello Miss Idaho! Sorry, but what's your first name?" As much as I enjoy being "the diabetic beauty queen", there's a lot more to me that I sometimes feel is ignored and forgotten.

Okay! Enough about us and our sadness! The more time I spend with the diabetes community, the more I grow to love you all. My heart is always full when I come home from a conference or camp, and I start counting down the days until the events that follow. I hope I always feel that way, and I deeply admire those who have dedicated a huge portion of their lives to supporting PWDs (person/people with diabetes), as well as finding a cure. Who knows if I will enjoy my involvement forever, or if I will continue to have little burnout periods. The reason I bring this up is, first and foremost, because I want you to be aware of it, and know that if you sometimes feel the same way, that's okay! I have definitely felt guilty about wanting to take a break from talking about diabetes, but after finding out that others definitely feel the same exact way as I do sometimes, I realized it's a natural (and acceptable) feeling to have. In her book *Raising Teens With Diabetes*, Moira McCarthy stresses the importance of talking to your teen with T1D while making decisions about whether to participate in diabetes service, namely, advocacy:

"Deciding to become an advocate is an important decision that teens and their parents need to think over carefully. If you've stepped up before and are considering it now, you and your teen will want to talk over all sides of it. And if you've long been a parent advocate along with a child who did a lot in preteen years, it's important you visit the topic with you teen now. Not all teens want to be active and visible in the diabetes advocacy world. Even if your teen loved it as a smaller child, you'll want to gauge his or her interest in it and feelings about it at this time, to be sure you are not pushing the teen into a place or movement he or she doesn't want to be a part of right now."

That being said, becoming involved with and making a difference in your local diabetes community can be extremely rewarding, and even bring you joy out of an otherwise depressing situation. It's also nice to escape once in awhile, though. As I said earlier, when we get together as fellow diabetics, it's not always for the purpose of talking about our diabetes, but rather to be with people who are exactly like you in order to avoid talking about it or answering questions from strangers. Adolescence is an especially hard time for teens to be different from their peers. We often wish we could remove "diabetic" from the list of adjectives that describe us. I bring this up just to make sure you are aware that if you or your child (if you are a parent of a T1D) seem burnt out on your current diabetes activities—whether it be full-time advocacy, walks for a cure, or a support group—that it is completely okay to take a break...which leads me to our final "universal" sugar linings: compassion and empathy.

13: Compassion and Empathy: My Other Storm Cloud

We all have many clouds, and diabetes is definitely not my only one. At some point in our lives, we will all face judgment, tragedy, and hardship. To say the least, facing each can be extremely painful. Looking at the bright side of an awful situation is the last thing we feel like doing when all we want to do is cry, grieve, or just be angry about whatever injustice has occurred. As I have said before, some clouds are larger and stormier than others and they can sometimes do a great job of hiding the sugar linings that lie behind them. I am grateful that I have been able to find many sugar linings from my diabetes, but all of our journeys are different, and yours may be more difficult and trying than mine has.

As it turns out, I have another major cloud in my life. It has been a larger, greyer, and more painful cloud than my diabetes. It hasn't brought any friends into my life—in fact, it has driven some away. I don't even really know if it's made me stronger. I have struggled with it my entire life, from the day I was born, and have been hurt by other people's judgments on a regular basis because of it.

Similar to the misinformed questions and comments we receive for having diabetes, people often don't understand, or make an attempt to understand, how I feel. I recently wrote a blog post about this ugly storm cloud in my life. It doesn't have much to do with diabetes, but the lesson I learned from this experience revealed a new sugar lining from my diabetes experience that I had never appreciated before:

April 6th, 2015

"I speak all over the country about the importance of loving who we are, and emphasize appreciating the things that make us feel different and self-conscious. They make us unique. Not only should we tolerate and not try to hide them, but instead celebrate and learn to love them. The world would be boring if we were all exactly the same. Diversity is wonderful, stimulating, and makes the world interesting. Yet, we have a slight fear of, and feel uncomfortable with, things that make the people around us seem foreign. Whether it is a difference in physical appearance, culture/religion, sexual orientation, or the fact that someone has a disability or maybe struggles with a mental health problem. That fear causes us to judge others, and that judgment is sometimes cruel and is always unnecessary. It is not our place to share our negative opinion about

other people just being themselves, even if it does make us uncomfortable. Those comments from others are exactly what cause each of us to think that something is wrong with who we are or what we look like.

"Lately, I have been feeling like a hypocrite. I have a secret—one that I am beyond ashamed of and never would have dreamed about sharing. I hate it. I sometimes hate myself because of it. After my speeches about self-esteem, I kick myself over not taking my own advice: love yourself. Love what makes you different. Be proud of being weird. At my high points, and actually the majority of the time, I do love myself. However, at those times, I love myself in spite of this insecurity, rather than because of it. Unlike realizing that my insulin pump totally rocks because I've used it to inspire other people, and that my shame about being talented "only" at math and science, and being secretly obsessed with reading as an adolescent (rather than the "cool" stuff, like sports, singing, art, dancing, and whatever else my peers seemed to excel at) was silly because in real life after high school, those are the talents that really matter, I hate this other specific insecurity and don't know if I will ever learn to love it. I've learned to laugh at the things make me a little weird, like my hands that are too big or that my nose wrinkles way too much when I laugh, but I can barely tolerate or accept the thing I have been trying to hide since I was born.

"Something that is encouraged in the diabetes community is to not hide the disease. Many times kids do not want their peers, or even teachers, to know. In my experience, I have found that in settings like that, where I have a small amount of anxiety about people looking at me weird, I find that I can actually attract less attention to my diabetes if everyone is aware of it. My friends and family have become blind to my pump, and when my glucometer beeps loudly with a result, they no longer notice, as it has become white noise to them. They are used to me eating at strange, otherwise seemingly inappropriate times. On the other hand, those things are all odd to those who are not aware that I have type one. So, in the hope that sharing about this, I will receive less hurtful comments, questions, and stares, I am writing this.

"It is difficult to hide my biggest insecurity. Actually, it's impossible. If you have spent an extended period of time with me, you most likely already know about it, but unless you are a family member or inseparable best friend, you may not understand it.

I have an eating disorder.

"It's not anorexia or bulimia. It is an involuntary eating disorder that is not at all based on body image. I eat plenty of calories. I love my body. I love it when it's Miss America ready, and I even love it when my tummy is poochy after stuffing my face with carbs, when my skin is a mixture of blinding whiteness and red blotchiness instead of spray tanned, when I am make-up free, and when I'm breaking out. Because, guess what? Despite the fact that I am a "beauty queen", it is nowhere in my job description to be anyone's eye candy. It is, however, encouraged for us to be confident and love how we look, even at our "worst", and set an example for girls that there are much more important things about us than our appearance. Anyone who bases his or her opinion of me on my appearance is not worth my time or energy. There is nothing about my body or physical appearance that I would ever change to make others happy. Some personality traits and habits, on the other hand, I wish I could.

"I do not have an eating disorder because I hate myself; however, I [sometimes] hate myself because I have an eating disorder. I suffer from SED, which stands for Selective Eating Disorder. It is has recently been changed officially to ARFID: Avoidant Restrictive Food Intake Disorder. The disorder is often mistaken for simply picky or fussy eating (which is a choice), and because of that, people are relentlessly cruel, disgusted by the thought of a 21-year-old woman acting like a spoiled child. Picky or fussy eating is a normal part of child development, and is grown out of once one has reached adulthood. ARFID, on the other hand, is a mental disorder involving a phobia of foods, flavors, and textures that is not outgrown and can be linked to other medical issues or disorders. It can cause lack of nutrition, and also severe anxiety and depression.

"Throughout my life, and still today, it is nearly impossible for anyone to take my disorder seriously. I did not even know it was a problem others also faced until I got past the age at which it was appropriate to be picky. After I discovered that I was not the only person in the world with this issue, and that other people also have the same disorder, I quickly found reassurance online from other adults who reported mainly eating grilled cheese sandwiches, pancakes, chicken nuggets (sound familiar close friends?), and other mildly flavored and tamely textured and flavored

Normal Picky Eating	Selective Eating Disorder
Onset - around 18 mos - 3 yrs	Onset - typically birth to age 4
usually accepts 30 or more foods	usually accepts less than 20 foods
choice, control	fear, anxiety
prefers a specific food for a long period of time	often rejects entire food - groups - (usually meat and/or vegetables)
typically has no medical issues	often associated with OCD, ASD, food trauma, oral-motor delay, swallowing disorder, SPD, or gastrointestinal disorders
typical sensory experiences	often repulsed by texture, taste smell and/or food touching
grows out of picky phase usually before age 6	can persist into adulthood. Eating socially is extremely stressful and often avoided.
will eat in response to hunger	refuses unfamiliar foods despite hunger
... is a normal part of childhood development	... is an eating disorder

Intended only to illustrate the differences between typical toddler pickiness and disordered picky eating in teens and adults. Not all examples are present in every individual with SED. Symptoms vary from person to person. Always seek a formal medical diagnosis from your primary healthcare provider.

photo credit: MealTimeHostage.com

"children's" foods that make up the majority of my diet. ARFID was added to the DSM-V (Diagnostic and Statistical Manual of Mental Disorders), which brought me even more peace knowing that experts in eating disorders were able to differentiate between simple picky eating and the disorder I have suffered from since I was born.

"(Here are links to more information on the disorder and stories of other people who also suffer from SED/ARFID: Kayleigh Roberts, Mealtime Hostage Blog, The Center for Eating Disorders (with info from the DSM-V), Ella Minker, No Thyself Blog (anonymous), and if you are still interested, ask Google. :D)

-note to reader: obviously, I could not provide links in a paper book, but you can view the original post at SierraSandison.org.

"Most comments, especially from people who spend the most time with me, are concerned about my nutrition. I understand that and appreciate that you care about me. However, I have had to answer questions about it my entire life, and my conversation with you (SURPRISE) is not the first time I have been told what eating healthy food means. Wait, you mean it's important to get protein and vegetables into my diet??? I had NO IDEA! Thank you so much!

"Okay, sorry about that. I have been thinking it inside my head for the past 21 years, and figured I would get out that sass while it isn't directed at a specific individual.

"I, obviously as someone who as competed in pageants with a swimsuit portion, care about my health and staying fit and in shape. Unlike other eating disorders, which are usually based on trying to lose weight, people ARFID struggle with fitting things into their diet that are not purely made of carbs. They can suffer from being overweight, due to the unhealthy foods they prefer (they are usually bread based). They can also suffer from not weighing enough because of avoiding food in any social situation. As someone who travels a lot, eating healthy is nearly impossible, and my priority then honestly is to just find something that will give me energy throughout the day. When I am at home, however, I get creative to make sure I am getting as much nutrients as I possibly can. It is a challenge. Most vegetables, and pretty much all fruits, have flavors that I can tolerate, and even enjoy. Their textures, on the other hand, trigger uncontrollable gag reflexes and my body will not accept them. In order to get my fruits and vegetables, I make fruit and veggie smoothies on a regular basis. "Haters", take note: whether they are liquid or in their traditional solid state, all that matters is that they get into my body (a fact that people don't really like to accept for some reason). The strides I have to go to in order

to stay healthy are weird, untraditional, and embarrassing. I hide them. I dread discussing them. They are also not anyone's business except mine, my parents', and my doctor's.

"The greatest challenge while living with ARFID is having to eat in social settings. Whether I have an empty plate, one with a few chips, rolls, or whatever the single item on the menu is that I am not afraid of, or have brought my own grilled cheese or peanut butter sandwich making supplies, I stand out. Questions are inevitable. Even when delivered in the kindest, most innocent way, they still crush me. All I want is to be able to eat and have everyone around be blind to the fact that I am not eating what they are: to completely ignore it; to not feel the urge to point it out; to let me just be me, sans judgmental curiosity. I will answer any question on diabetes. I am fine discussing politics and religion all night long. I die of embarrassment when I am forced to talk about food. I beg you, please do not make me. Please ignore it. I experience extreme anxiety for hours, sometimes even days, leading up to banquets that I am hired to speak at, dinners at new boyfriends' houses for the first time, and even at family reunions with cousins who resent that I, unlike them, am not grounded for not eating my green beans, and therefore don't let me forget how awful of a person I am for being different.

"There is no treatment for ARFID since it is rare and just recently recognized as a legitimate disorder. The most important things while managing it are: 1) trying to be as creative as possible in maintaining a healthy diet and 2) managing the, often extreme, anxiety and depression that it causes (due to social situations, and also traumatic encounters with foreign foods). Again, unlike picky eating, ARFID is not a choice. I would never, ever choose to live with this disorder. I wish everyday that I could change. If you insist on telling me that you still believe it's a choice, please save your breath and keep your comments to yourself.

"I am writing this because of a last-straw incident that, like basically every other time I have had to eat socially, ended in tears, suicidal thoughts, a revival of self-hatred, and my heart being shattered. I am hoping, like when sharing about my diabetes, that the people who care about me will remember this the next time we are eating together. Even if you don't care about me, please find an ounce of empathy in your heart to let me feel normal for once.

"I have made a list of the comments and "frequently asked questions" that I encounter in almost every social eating environment, please excuse any comments that sound harsh. I have 21 years of hurt and bitterness built up.

"ARFID Don'ts:

"(note: the harsh tone isn't aimed at you, the reader, so please excuse my sassy/mean venting)

- *Do not blame my parents.*

"I can handle getting picked on and judged myself. It sucks, but I have to deal with it everyday. What really puts me over the edge is when someone says, "isn't your dad a doctor?", "why haven't you parents taught you how to eat healthy?", "that would never, ever fly in our household. We tell our kids that they eat what they are given, or they starve." Comments like those don't just hurt, they infuriate me.

"How dare you? How **DARE** *you?! I have the greatest parents in the world. They recognized that I had something much more serious than a typical child's picky eating. A common sign, and huge issue, with living with ARFID is that we will actually choose to starve before putting something in our mouths that we are terrified of. Experts think that this is usually, but not always, caused by traumatic food experiences in early childhood, which leads me to the next reason my parents realized they shouldn't force me to eat anything: the vomiting and gag flexes that were triggered when they did. And, like good parents should, they didn't let me starve. They don't mock me in public eating settings. They help me avoid*

them when possible. They respectfully explain to hosts about my disorder so they are not shocked or surprised when I don't put much on my plate. They tell me to ignore people who judge me and do not understand, and they do what they can to make sure we figure out ways for me to eat as healthily as I possibly can.

- Lecture me on my nutrition.

"Thank you for caring. I really do appreciate it if you are not asking questions in a condescending way. However, I am already aware that I need protein, fruits, and veggies in my diet. I will take care of my body; you take care of yours.

- Attempt to force me into to trying new foods.

"First of all, 99% of the time you will not succeed. If you persist, I will most likely break off our friendship because of how uncomfortable I feel. I have even ended romantic relationships because of it. It is a phobia, and people with ARFID starve over eating something their body won't accept. Breaking off relationships is nothing compared to starvation.

- Succeed at forcing me into trying new foods.

"If you do manage to get me to put something in my mouth, I really hope it is not something you cooked yourself, because the vomiting that inevitably follows may offend you. A sign of ARFID is avoiding trying new foods at all costs, especially when we are not in private, because we know the consequences of putting the food into our mouths is much worse than not attempting to at all.

• Talk about it to other people—both behind my back and in my earshot.

"The exception to this is if you are my parents, boyfriend, best friend, or manager/event coordinator, and I have asked you to let people know ahead of time to please not mention any weird eating behaviors of mine during an event I have had extreme anxiety about.

• Tell me you think it is a choice.

"You are not me. You do not understand my mind. Please study the meaning of "empathy." If I could change, I would in a heart beat. That has always been my answer to, "if a genie gave you 1 wish, what would you ask for?" I want to be normal. And, hypothetically, if it were a choice, it is my body. It being a choice would still not give you any right to treat me cruelly or judge me. If you lack any empathy towards my condition, than I highly doubt you are genuinely concerned about my health or nutrition.

• Tell me I am missing out on "so many wonderful foods."

"I am terrified of food. I despise flavor. Please respect that.

- *Warn me that there will be many social gatherings in the future that I will need to eat food at.*

"There have also been many social gatherings involving food in my past. I am more aware of this than you will ever know. Thank you for the reminder. Please keep it to yourself.

- *Laugh at me at a restaurant as I order a grilled cheese off the kids' menu.*

"I am fully aware of the fact that I am a 21-year-old woman. It's not funny. It's embarrassing.

- *Don't tell people I "don't eat anything".*

"I eat a lot—in quantity, not variety—you just don't see it. Eating disorders already have a negative connotation; please do not embarrass me more than I already am.

"I am sorry for my harsh, sassy tone above. Now, if you have read this far, it is clear that you really do care about me and want to better understand the condition that you have so many questions about. Here are a couple more don'ts, that don't make me angry, but I want you to know about:

- *Please don't feel bad if you invite me to a dinner party and there is no food for me to eat. I really am used to it, and will eat before or after. My anxiety doesn't lie in not having something to eat at an event, it lies in people commenting on it being burdened by my disorder. Please, don't worry about me. I will be fine, and will just be grateful you invited me and didn't comment about the fact that I'm not eating.*

- *Please don't choose a restaurant based on making sure they have something for me on the menu. Seriously, as long as no one comments on the fact that I didn't get anything, I sometimes appreciate having an excuse to not spend money on eating out.*

"All I really want is to be able to go to social events without having to be noticed (in a negative way), judged, or question. The best thing to do is just ignore me. If I really need something, I will ask. If in doubt about whether I will be comfortable with a question or comment you have, either don't ask, or ask me in a setting in which I am not expected to eat.

Finally, another reason I decided to write this and "come out of the pantry" is that part of the depression that follows a social event (such as the recent incident) includes, again, kicking myself over the fact that I travel the country telling kids to not only tolerate, but love the things that make them different. Yet here I am, beating myself up over my eating disorder. I don't think I will ever love it. Unlike with my diabetes diagnosis, and all the wonderful things that came out of it, I would wish my ARFID and my entire experience with it away in a millisecond if I could.

"What I have learned is that sometimes, the good things that come out of the obstacles in life are not always great enough to make the bad experience worth it. Nothing replaces a lost loved one. Nothing can take back the damage of a traumatic or abusive childhood. I don't think anything will make me feel as if my eating disorder has been completely worth it. However, I do believe that there is always a silver lining in every situation, even if it is teeny tiny, and it is always worth looking for in order to make the experience slightly less miserable.

"I have never seen a silver lining in my eating disorder until this last traumatic event, but I think I have finally found it.

"Living with this disorder that so many people insist is a choice, and painfully knowing the truth that they will never accept, has given me a great ability to empathize. There will be people I meet with differences that I don't, and can't, fully understand. I know what it's like to have people refuse to listen to me, not accept me for who I am, and mercilessly berate me. If nothing else good ever comes out of living with this disorder, I know I will always do my best to never, ever be one of those people who judge too quickly because it is not my place, and I have never walked in the other person's shoes. I hope that I will never make a comment that is cruel or hurts someone's feelings about something that they can't help. I will keep the pain I have felt in mind when I see a child misbehaving and feel irritated with his parents; we may not see it, but he may suffer from autism or some other mental or social disorder. I will remember what it feels like to be judged the next time I see a homeless person. I do not know their story. I will never blame an obese person for their weight problems by assuming their weight is their fault or due to laziness. Empathy and compassion are the most important values I have, and if my disorder helps to better exemplify them, I am grateful.

"Thank you for reading this if you have gotten this far. It would really mean the world if even one person took the time to better understand my condition. Xoxo."

Soon after I posted this link to the blog on Facebook, unexpected support and love came pouring in. I noticed a common theme in the comments: my followers with diabetes understood how I felt better than anyone else.

Living with diabetes teaches us what it's like to be judged and hurt by the misinformed comments that we hear way too often. We know how it feels when someone stares at our pump or gets uncomfortable around a needle. People jump to conclusions and are eager to blame us for causing our autoimmune disease by eating too much junk food or not exercising enough.

We know all too well what it's like to receive the uncomfortable questions and judgmental glances. We also know what a relief it is to find a friend who understands exactly how we feel. How often do we wish that other people could walk in our shoes, just for a day, to understand what it's like to live with diabetes?

There are people in your life who feel the same way about whatever their cloud may be, wishing daily that the ones around them could understand. Even though there is no way to switch lives with them, we still have tasted the same feelings they are experiencing: feeling different, misunderstood, and judged; facing hurtful comments, pain, and adversity.

We have a choice to either ignore their similarities, and be the person who casts judgment, *or* to use our experience with diabetes to better understand and empathize with them—to be the friend that others so desperately need, and that we often wish for. Be the latter.

Sometimes (more often than not, really) sugar linings like to hide. If you are having an especially difficult time in your diabetes journey, and are having trouble finding a sugar lining, start with finding empathy and compassion for others who are also struggling to find their bright side.

Some of the trials we face in our life, as well as the insecurities we might have, can seem so awful that there may not be much of a bright side. In those situations, we can at least still remember what it felt like. Even if it is different from what others may be going through, we still know what it's like to experience pain and judgment. As I said at the beginning of my blog post, diversity is so powerful! Being unique is awesome! Unfortunately, we have a natural tendency to be uncomfortable with things that seem foreign and different.

The next time you feel tempted to judge someone, or jump to conclusions about their situation, remember what it feels like when someone else does the same to you. Stop yourself, and don't be the insensitive person that causes pain to others. The fact is, most people struggle with self-esteem. We are socialized to think that being different is bad. We have a fear of the unknown. We also fear judgment. I know that, if nothing else, the trials I have faced in my life have given me a greater ability to empathize with others and be compassionate. Be open-minded. Be accepting. Try your best to love others, even if you don't fully understand the things that make them different from you.

14: Finding and Sharing *Your* Sugar Linings

Throughout this book, I have focused on my own personal story, along with four sugar linings that seem to be true for almost all people living with type 1: strength, friendship, service, and, finally, a greater ability to show compassion and empathy towards others.

While traveling, I have heard stories from many different people who live with type 1, and, inevitably, they have shared some other unique (and sometimes silly) sugar linings that make living with their disease more tolerable and, sometimes, even enjoyable. I love hearing about them!

One of the most popular diabetes bloggers, Kim Vlasnik (who I mentioned in the DiaBesties Chapter) from TextingMyPancreas.com, made a video called *The Bright Side*. My favorite thing she mentions? Using test strips as teeny tiny bookmarks.

Whether the sugar linings you find are life changing (such as strength or a priceless friendship), or awesome and silly (such as using your test strips as little bookmarks), I encourage you to always be looking for them. When you find them, cherish them.

You should also share them! We are all in this together. If you have some sugar linings in mind that you've found relating to your diabetes or anything else in your life (and if you ever come across any in the future) that I haven't mentioned, I want to hear about them! On August 1st, 2015, I will be launching The Sugar Linings Blog, which I will use to document my journey with diabetes from here on out. Most importantly, it will focus on the stories you submit, discussing the bright side (and sometimes, the not-so-bright side, since we need to vent sometimes) of your experience with diabetes!

We want to hear from people who live with diabetes, as well as parents, siblings, spouses, and friends of those living with the disease. I would also love to hear the stories of people who have gone through different adversities—other than T1D—who want to share the bright side they found from their own difficult experiences.

How have YOU found your own sugar linings? Let me know by going to TheSugarLiningsBlog.com or by emailing sugarliningsblog.com! You can also follow me: @sierrasandison. Tweet me your sugar linings, tag me in a picture on Instagram with you and your DiaBestie, and follow me on Facebook at facebook.com/sierrasandison to keep in touch with me!

Speaking of which, I have two favors to ask you:

1) If you enjoyed my book, it would be a HUGE help if you went on Amazon and left a review! (And of course, recommend the book to your T1D friends who may benefit from it).

2) Take a picture of you and your copy of Sugar Linings and post it on Twitter or Instagram with the #showmeyourbook, and tag me, @sierrasandison, for a RT (and maybe even a follow) ;D

I hope I have been able to bring some light into a seemingly dark and gloomy forecast, and that it is just the beginning of the light and sugar linings the blog will bring in the future! Also make sure to check out the resources I have provided on the blog to help you get plugged into the "#DOC" (Diabetes Online Community). I have listed some of my favorite bloggers, Facebook book pages, Instagram accounts, and other awesome diabetes online resources, which have helped me get through the toughest seasons of my own disease. Whether it is to ask questions, get advice, find some occasional humor in the disease, or just to connect with people who will listen and know exactly how you're feeling, the DOC is an amazing and supportive community to be a part of.

• • •

Living with a chronic, incurable disease is...well, not always fun, to say the least. Right now, we can't make our diabetes go away or reverse the damage it may have already inflicted on our bodies. However, we can believe that there is a plan for our lives, as well as sugar linings waiting to be found behind every cloud that may enter our lives. Be ready to find them when the forecast starts to look bleak. They are there!

Whatever hardship you are facing in life, I believe that a sugar lining can be found, even if it may be small. Your bright side may be the strength and resilience your situation has brought you, or the friendships that have grown out of it with people who are in similar circumstances. It may give you a way to make a difference, and will definitely help you understand and be more compassionate towards others who are struggling. I hope that at least one (but hopefully all) of these holds true for you, and maybe even other sugar linings that I haven't experienced or even thought of!

Finally, I want you to take pride in what you have already endured. Whether you are a parent of a PWD, a PWD yourself, or instead, have a cloud that has nothing to do with type 1 diabetes, I know you have overcome a lot. If you were diagnosed just yesterday, you have already made it twenty-four hours. Sometimes that first day or first week is the most difficult. Surviving it is something to be proud of. Several times in this book, I have mentioned how I sometimes question whether I have avoided letting diabetes takeover my identity. I hear over and over again, "don't let diabetes define you," and "you are so much more than your disease." Yet, to most, that is the only thing they know about me. Have I failed at following those commands to keep my disease out of my identity? I recently wrote a blog post that mentioned the feelings I have had in the past, and Mark B. left this kind comment:

"Sierra, when on those bad days you feel that, to many, you are the diabetic beauty queen, I'm going to ask you to find a sense of pride. That pageant win was inspirational for so many of us t1ds. Type 1 had a way of ruining our plans way too much. Coming down from a high for over two hours means I didn't get to play volleyball with my friends. Volleyball is one of the best ways I have to stay in shape. I may get a little low, but it's simple and I don't crash. Recovery from a low that takes 45 minutes can mean that I miss a

movie or some other plan because I should've left a half hour ago. I don't let these things beat me, but I get frustrated when they ruin part of my day. Your winning that crown after sporting your pump just raises our determination a few notches. While we may refer to you as the diabetic beauty queen, it is done with pride. It's like someone from our family did it. We know the hurdles that we go through, and we understand that you probably have dealt with many of the same hurdles. I know the planning that goes into a two-day trip an hour and a half away. I see pictures of you going overseas and think, "yeah, I'm going to do that". While t1d may take some of your identity, you have taken it back, with interest. Thank you for seeing that pageant all the way to its conclusion, and own everything about it with strength and inspiration. That's what "the diabetic beauty queen" means to many t1ds!"

I believe I have come to terms with the fact that being so involved with diabetes activities does not mean that diabetes has taken over my identity. While I don't love my disease, I love the people I meet who also live with it, the opportunities that have come from it, and the pride that I have in having managed this disease for over three years now. Maybe diabetes is a part of my identity that I have to live with. But what I have done with it, and the way I have not let it hold me back these past three years, is something I have become extremely proud of. Diabetes is not my identity; being someone who is kicking its butt is.

. . .

Life gives no one immunity against adversity, but life gives to everyone the power of positive thought, which is sufficient to master all circumstances of adversity and convert them into benefits.

~Napoleon Hill

For the first year or so after being diagnosed, I told myself everyday that the fateful day after my snowboarding trip was the worst day of my life. I looked back with bitterness, remembering the times before where I would go to the movies and stuff my face with popcorn, or eat a tub of cookie dough with my best friend as we watched Netflix and my body would digest the food on its own. I had no clue as to how many carbs the food contained, nor did I care. I took my body's ability to turn food into energy for granted. Why couldn't I return to those days? Why?!

Since that day, I have experienced many highs and lows (literally). I have walked on the Miss America stage, and felt that that moment alone was worth everything I had gone through. I have found best friends that now mean the world to me. I have learned to love others deeper and to put much more effort into attempting to understand their pain. I have also had to deal with miserable out-of-range blood sugars, and too many needles to count. When my body decides it doesn't want to cooperate with me on any given day, it can ruin plans with friends, make me late to work, or completely put me out of commission. I've had to deal with the misinformed comments and hurtful questions that most PWDs have to hear many times throughout their life.

Of course, I am thankful for my sugar linings, but I've also recently realized that I am grateful for all of the low points as well. Why the heck would I be grateful for the negative side of diabetes, you ask? Diabetes is the storm cloud that the majority of us (you, I, and the rest of the readers) share. Whether or not you or a loved one live with diabetes, you have, at some point in your life, faced hardship. Diabetes is just one of the multiple clouds we will encounter throughout our lives. I have had many difficult times in my past, and I know I will also have adversities come up in my future. The negative and difficult side of diabetes has made me stronger and has better prepared me to face the storm clouds that, without a doubt, lie ahead for me.

Today, I look back at that day I was diagnosed with much less bitterness. I still hate my disease, but I am also grateful for the things it has taught me, and the wonderful people it has brought into my life. I have learned to make spending time and energy focusing on the positive an important part of my diabetes management routine. It has made all the difference. I realize that even though my diabetes has come along with much pain and frustration, I now consider that day as one of the most important days of my life.

Going forward, diabetes equips us for future clouds by helping us develop greater resilience and perseverance. We are strong enough to have survived diabetes so far, so we know that we can get through whatever life throws at us next. Most importantly, we are aware that looking for sugar linings in difficult situations is not only possible, but also an important part of getting through our greatest struggles.

You are strong. You have shown incredible resilience and perseverance. You have made it this far. Some of you have probably done things you never dreamed you could do without diabetes, let alone with it. You haven't let diabetes stop you. Be proud of what you have overcome. Press on, even on the days where your blood sugar is uncooperative and you feel like giving up. You may not have the ability to produce your own insulin, but, as Napoleon Hill said, you *do* have the "power of positive thought." Make time to look for a bright side of your diagnosis and cherish the sugar linings that come along with your cloud every chance you get: they are there.

Acknowledgments

In the process of writing this book, I have spent the [many] days that I suffered from writer's block reading books on how to write and market a book. In almost all of them, the author expressed their struggles with self-doubt. I came up with the concept of sugar linings forever ago, but never actually opened my laptop to start typing. Who would read what I had to say? Who cared? Would the concept of sugar linings be controversial? I want to be sensitive to other peoples' pain and adversities. How will I write this book without seeming like I am trying to discredit or belittle the suffering that diabetes causes them? That isn't my intention at all! So, for months the book remained a vague idea, existing solely in my mind. Hadley George, my DiaBestie that you learned about earlier in this book, lives in Ohio and is one of the few people I am completely honest with about my feelings and frustrations with diabetes (until now, as I publish this book and spill my heart out to you). During my last trip to Cincinnati, I mentioned the book to Hadley, and her excitement about the idea gave me the courage to finally start plunking away on my keyboard. Thank you so much, Hads! Without you believing in and encouraging me, this book would have forever lived in my mind, instead of on paper (or kindle, as I prefer).

McCall Salinas, you are like the little sister I wish I had: one that I never fight with, thinks I am the coolest person on the planet, and never steals my clothes. (Hailey and Sydney: take note. Also, I want my brand new dress back!)

It's an incredible feeling to have someone look up to me, especially when my confidence is lacking or I begin to wonder if all my hard work is even making a difference. I am so proud of the woman you are becoming, and I can't wait to watch you grow up even more (and change the world while you're at it)!

I want to thank my wonderful boyfriend, Brendon Smith, who is very gracious in dealing with me being out-of-state more often than not and picking me up and dropping me off from the airport at ungodly hours several times a week. I am extremely grateful for and proud of your artistic talent, and the hours you spent designing multiple options for my book cover. When I feel discouraged, or when my fear of failure rears its ugly head, you have constantly given me a reminder of the support and love I have received from the diabetes community when I needed it most, leading up to my book publishing. Most importantly, thank you for loving me (insulin pump and all), always being more responsible than me by keeping track of my Dexcom, getting orange juice whenever I need it, being the BEST ADVENTURE (AND LIFE) BUDDY EVER, and being a wonderful/my favorite human. I love you so much.

Thank you to my dad for reading this book approximately 10 million times before I handed it off to an editor, and for raising me to look for my sugar linings.

Thank you to everyone who makes the Miss Idaho Organization, Miss America Organization, Miss Magic Valley, and Miss Pocatello Organizations possible, as well as my Miss Idaho judges, and Nicole Johnson for believing in, encouraging, and inspiring me. You made this journey possible and my dream come true. I am eternally grateful.

Finally, thank you to everyone who has expressed excitement and support leading up to my publishing date. I have discovered that publishing a book can be a scary and vulnerable experience. Whenever I doubt myself, my heart is instantly filled back up when I hear or read your supportive and loving comments.

About the Author

While Sierra was growing up, she struggled with her self-esteem and trying to fit in, as well as with finding her identity. After being diagnosed with type 1 diabetes at the age of 18, she hated her disease—not only because it was affecting her health, but also because of how it made her feel more different than she already was. She refused to wear an insulin pump until she heard about Nicole Johnson, Miss America 1999. Nicole, who also lives with T1D, quickly became Sierra's hero. Nicole's example helped Sierra develop an empowering confidence, which transformed her life. Sierra made it her goal to some day wear an insulin pump while competing on the Miss America stage in order to do for others what Nicole Johnson had done for her. Less than three years later, she achieved her dream, along with launching the viral #showmeyourpump campaign which encouraged diabetics worldwide to proudly show their insulin pumps on social media. Since then, Sierra has appeared on the Dr. Oz Show, the cover of *Diabetes Forecast* magazine, and Good Morning America. She now spends her time speaking at schools, diabetes conferences, and other events across the country. She tells her story, along with the message of overcoming adversity, and loving the things that make you unique, rather than being ashamed of the things that make you different. Now, with the launch of her new book, *Sugar Linings: Finding the Bright Side of Type 1 Diabetes*, she hopes to send a new message: one of hope and encouragement for diabetics and non-diabetics alike.

@sierrasandison | @sierrasandison | facebook.com/sierrasandison

If you are interested in hiring Sierra to speak at your next event, go to SierraSandison.org for more information on scheduling and prices.